Compendium of HIV Prevention Interventions with Evidence of Effectiveness

from
CDC's HIV/AIDS Prevention Research Synthesis Project

November 1999 (Revised on August 31, 2001)

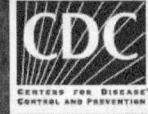

Compendium of HIV Prevention Interventions with Evidence of Effectiveness

from
CDC's HIV/AIDS
Prevention Research Synthesis Project

Centers for Disease Control and Prevention
National Center for HIV, STD, and TB Prevention
Division of HIV/AIDS Prevention - Intervention Research and Support
Atlanta, Georgia

November 1999
Revised

Acknowledgments

Many individuals, groups, organizations, and communities contributed to this *Compendium*. We are most grateful to those who participated in the research studies. They trusted that their time and effort in a study would increase our understanding about ways to prevent HIV/AIDS. We hope this document confirms their trust and supports their prevention goals.

Similarly, we thank the researchers who designed the interventions and carried out the studies. In the course of writing this document, we spoke with many of the original researchers. Their contact information throughout the *Compendium* underscores their continued commitment to HIV/AIDS prevention.

For the selection of effective interventions by applying consistent criteria, thanks to John Anderson, Wayne D. Johnson, Linda Kay, Mary Neumann, Salaam Semaan, and Ellen Sogolow of the Centers for Disease Control and Prevention (CDC); Don Des Jarlais of Beth Israel Medical Center; and Larry Hedges of the University of Chicago. For reviews of drafts and comments that improved the final document, thanks to Amy DeGroff, Nikki Economou, Michele Evering-Watley, Dorothy Gunther, Lynn Meinor, John Peppert, Lauretta Pinckney, Tamara Sloan-Anderson, Kathy Stark, Chris Tullier, Duane Wilkerson, and Mary Willingham.

Special acknowledgments go to the project leadership and staff of CDC's contractor, Aspen Systems Corporation, particularly Ruthann Bates, Meredith Hart, Kevin Hylton, Maryann Krayer, Paula Lipman, Sarah McClanahan, and Darcy Strouse. At CDC, special thanks to Bobbie Person and Linda Kay for leadership with the earlier drafts and the later drafts, respectively. Lynda Doll's suggestions at several stages strengthened both scientific soundness and clarity.

Suggested Citation: Centers for Disease Control and Prevention, HIV/AIDS Prevention Research Synthesis Project. Compendium of HIV Prevention Interventions with Evidence of Effectiveness. Atlanta, GA: Centers for Disease Control and Prevention; November 1999, Revised, [inclusive page numbers].

Contents

Drug Users

Heterosexual Adults

---

[1]ACDP and Magura include multiple target populations, however, their summaries appear only once.

[1] ACDP and Magura include multiple target populations, however, their summaries appear only once.

Alphabetical Listing of HIV Prevention Interventions:

[1]ACDP and Magura include multiple target populations, however, their summaries appear only once.

Introduction

The Centers for Disease Control and Prevention (CDC) developed this *Compendium of HIV Prevention Interventions with Evidence of Effectiveness* to respond to prevention service providers, planners, and others who request science-based interventions that work to prevent HIV transmission. All interventions selected for this *Compendium* came from behavioral or social studies that had both intervention and control/comparison groups and positive results for behavioral or health outcomes. We required designs with control/comparison groups so that successful results could be attributed to the interventions. Appendix A describes in detail the criteria used to select the interventions. This document provides *Summaries* of each intervention that met all criteria. These are referred to as effective interventions. To meet the ongoing need for current information about what works in HIV prevention, this *Compendium* will be updated periodically.

The *Compendium* provides state-of-the-science information about interventions with evidence of reducing sex- and/or drug-related risks, and the rate of HIV/STD infections. These interventions have been effective with a variety of populations, e.g., clinic patients, heterosexual men and women, high-risk youth, incarcerated populations, injection drug users, and men who have sex with men. They have been delivered to individuals, groups, and communities in settings such as storefronts, gay bars, health centers, housing communities, and schools.

A reader may want to consider an entire group of studies, for instance, all studies that used small group interventions. Table 1 highlights population and intervention characteristics for each of the interventions. Accessing additional materials may assist in implementing a selected intervention. Table 2 indicates the interventions that are part of CDC's Replicating Effective Programs (REP), Prevention Counseling Course Series, and Research to Classroom: Programs That Work (PTW) projects. These ongoing projects support development of intervention materials, training, and technical assistance.

Once an intervention is adopted, its actual impact will depend on how it is implemented. The important thing is to achieve a balance between adapting the intervention to suit local needs and maintaining the core elements and key characteristics that made the original intervention successful. Also, the agency that implements the intervention will require organizational support, adequate staffing, and sufficient resources for implementation.

Finally, some readers may prefer an alternative or additional approach. They may want to assess and strengthen their existing program activities rather than select a new intervention, or to do both. We offer an Intervention Checklist to guide this process. The items on the Checklist are derived from many successful prevention interventions.

How the *Compendium* Is Organized

The *Compendium* is organized into four sections:

Section One: Summaries of Prevention Interventions

This section provides "one-pagers" or *Summaries* of each effective intervention. These are written to emphasize the intervention content and methods, based on information provided in the report. *Summaries* are grouped by target populations:

| Drug Users | Heterosexual Adults | Men Who Have Sex With Men | 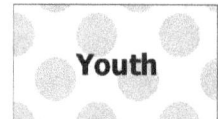 Youth |

Within groups, *Summaries* are ordered alphabetically by author.

Section Two: Tables

For all interventions, *Table 1* highlights characteristics of the populations and interventions.
For selected interventions, *Table 2* provides information about access to intervention materials.

Section Three: Intervention Checklist

The *Intervention Checklist* is a tool for intervention assessment. It is designed to clarify aspects of existing interventions that can be strengthened.

Section Four: Appendices

Appendix A describes the aims of CDC's HIV/AIDS Prevention Research Synthesis (PRS) project, the criteria used to select PRS relevant and rigorous studies, and the additional criteria used to select a subset of relevant and rigorous studies for the *Compendium*.

Appendix B contains the bibliography, which references each study in the *Compendium*, along with additional or supplemental citations that pertain to that study.

Section 1
Summaries of HIV Prevention Interventions

Summary Format

Section 1. Summaries of HIV Prevention Interventions uses a standard format, with the same elements used to describe each intervention. If an element is missing from a *Summary,* it is because the source citation does not contain that information. The following elements comprise the format:

Title, authors, reference -   bibliographic information for the source report (usually a journal publication, but may be "in press" or "submitted for publication")

Intervention goal(s) -   selected behavioral/health aims of the intervention (most often other aims exist but are outside the scope of the *Summary*)

Intervention setting -   the type of place in which the intervention was conducted

Population -   includes the following features:
    sample size -   the number of people who participated (usually the total number in the intervention and control conditions of the study at baseline)

    demographics -   selected characteristics of the participants (e.g., gender, race/ethnicity, age, education, income)

Comparison condition -   describes briefly what was provided to participants who did not receive the intervention during the study (e.g., a non-HIV intervention, usual HIV services such as HIV education and HIV counseling and testing)

Intervention description -   includes the following features:
    theory/model -   the basis for the design of the intervention, which explains the behavior change
    duration -   the length and number of intervention sessions
    location -   where the intervention was carried out
    facilitators/leader
    characteristics -   e.g., gender, race/ethnicity, age
    content -   e.g., topics, information, skills pertaining to risk reduction
    method(s) -   how the intervention was delivered or conducted
    handout(s) -   materials given to participants
    incentives -   cash/items used to encourage or support participation

Findings -   selected behavioral or health outcomes (usually at three or six months after intervention)

Contact person -   the research scientist (or designee) who conducted the intervention and/or its evaluation

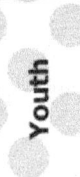

Youth

Men Who Have Sex With Men

Heterosexual Adults

Drug Users

Community-level HIV Intervention in Five Cities:Final Outcome Data from the CDC AIDS Community Demonstration Projects

CDC AIDS Community Demonstration Projects Research Group (1999)

American Journal of Public Health, 89 (3), 336 - 345

Intervention Goal(s): To determine the effects of a community-level intervention to increase condom use with main and non-main partners and/or to increase disinfection of injection equipment.

Intervention Setting: Street settings, public sex environments, and other community venues.

Description of Intervention: AIDS Community Demonstration Project

This community-level intervention was based on the Transtheoretical Model of Behavior Change, which recognizes that change occurs in stages. The intervention aimed to modify attitudes and beliefs about prevention methods among the community members by providing models of successful risk-reduction strategies adopted by members of the target population. The intervention took place over 3 years in Dallas, Denver, Long Beach, New York City, and Seattle. Peer volunteers from each target community were trained to carry out the intervention, drawing attention to and reinforcing identification with and acceptance of the intervention messages.

The intervention featured role model stories developed from the real-life experiences of local community members. These stories depicted members of the target population moving from earlier to later stages of change. Stories were developed and selected so that the majority matched the predominant stages of change and beliefs about condoms and bleach observed in the population.

The role model stories were featured in flyers distributed with condoms and bleach kits by the peer volunteers.

Population: Interviews were conducted with 15,205 individuals who were injection drug users, female sex partners of injection drug users, commercial sex workers, non-gay-identified men who have sex with men, high-risk youth, and/or residents in census tracts with high rates of sexually transmitted disease. Of the interviewees, 45% were men and 55% were women; 54% were African American, 19% were Hispanic, 22% were white, and 5% were of other racial/ethnic groups; and 35% were under 30 years of age.

Comparison Condition: Usual HIV prevention activities and services available in the community.

Behavioral/Health Findings: Individuals in the intervention communities demonstrated significantly greater achievement of consistent condom use and maintenance of consistent condom use with non-main partners than individuals in the comparison communities.

Contact:

Behavioral Intervention Research Branch
Division of HIV & AIDS Prevention
Centers for Disease Control and Prevention
Atlanta, GA 30333

Phone: 404-639-1900
Fax: 404-639-1950
E-mail: ryw1@cdc.gov

AIDS and the Transition to Illicit Drug Injection– Results of a Randomized Trial Prevention Program

Des Jarlais, D.C., Casriel, C., Friedman, S.R., & Rosenblum, A. (1992).

British Journal of Addiction 87 (3), 493 - 498

Intervention Goal(s): To determine the effects of a small group intervention to prevent the transition from sniffing heroin to injecting heroin.

Intervention Setting: Community storefront.[§]

Description of Intervention:
AIDS/Drug Injection Prevention

This prevention program was based on social learning principles. The intervention was delivered in four 1- to 1½-hour sessions over a 2-week time period. The intervention was led by two trainers who encouraged a therapeutic atmosphere in which participants felt free to discuss personal problem situations and seek help from the trainers and from their peers. Reduction in non-injected use of illicit drugs was an additional goal of the program. Trainers were clear not to take a condemning/punitive attitude. The emphasis was on recognizing and admitting problems with illicit drug use and then seeking treatment to reduce/eliminate the illicit drug use.

The four sessions covered understanding AIDS, risks of drug use and drug injection, sexual behavior and AIDS, and seeking entry into drug abuse treatment programs. The trainers used presentations, group discussion, and role-play of critical situations like refusing an offer of injection or seeking entry into a treatment program when one's non-injection drug use becomes too heavy.

Population: Of the 83 drug users (heroin sniffers) who participated in the study, 70% were men and 30% were women; 26% were African American, 23% were Hispanic, and 51% were white. The average age of the participants was 27 years.

Comparison Condition: AIDS information and HIV antibody pretest counseling (HIV test optional).

Behavioral/Health Findings: Men and women who participated in the intervention were significantly less likely to inject drugs than those in the comparison condition.

Contact:
Don C. Des Jarlais, PhD
Chemical Dependency Institute
Beth Israel Medical Center
1st Avenue at 16th Street
New York, NY 10003

Phone: 212–387–3803
Fax: 212–387–3897
E-mail: dcdesjarla@aol.com

§ Information obtained from related reports or author.

This study meets CDC's HIV/AIDS Prevention Research Synthesis project criteria for relevance and methodological rigor and also has the positive and significant behavioral/health findings required for the *Compendium*. Date added 1/99

1-3

15-month Follow-up of Women Methadone Patients Taught Skills to Reduce Heterosexual HIV Transmission

El-Bassel, N. & Schilling, R.F. (1992).

Public Health Reports, 107 (5), 500-504

Intervention Goal(s): To determine the effects of a small group intervention to reduce sexual risk behavior and HIV transmission by increasing AIDS knowledge, sexual negotiation skills, and safer sex practices.

Intervention Setting: Methadone maintenance clinics.

Description of Intervention: Skills Building

The intervention was delivered in five 2-hour sessions[§] with about ten women in each group. The intervention was led by experienced female drug counselors who had received an additional 20 hours of training.

Sessions 1-2: Information on AIDS transmission and prevention. Trainers used video, other visual presentations, and didactic exercises to enable participants to identify their own high-risk sexual behaviors and barriers to adopting safer sex practices.

Session 3: Condom use. Members discussed their negative associations with condoms, practiced condom skills, and role-played scenarios that involved asking their partners to use condoms.

Sessions 4-5: Assertiveness training, problem solving, and communication skills. Participants practiced and personalized these skills, first by role-playing in scripted scenarios, then by selecting scenarios that reflected their own life.

Incentives included modest payments for attending the sessions.

Population: Of the 84 female methadone patients who participated in the study, 36% were African American and 64% were Hispanic[§]. The average age of the women was 35 years, and 90% were unemployed.

Comparison Condition: HIV/AIDS information only.

Behavioral Findings: Women who participated in the intervention significantly increased frequency of condom use with their partners compared with women in the comparison condition.

Contact:
Nabila El-Bassel, DSW
Columbia University School of Social Work
622 West 113th Street
New York, NY 10025

Phone: 212-854-5011
Fax: 212-854-8549
E-mail: ne5@columbia.edu

§ Information obtained from related reports or author.

This study meets CDC's HIV/AIDS Prevention Research Synthesis project criteria for relevance and methodological rigor and also has the positive and significant behavioral/health findings required for the *Compendium*. Date added 1/99

Outcomes of Intensive AIDS Education for Male Adolescent Drug Users in Jail

Magura, S., Kang, S., & Shapiro, J.L. (1994).

Journal of Adolescent Health, 15 (6), 457 - 463

Intervention Goal(s): To determine the effects of a small group intervention to reduce HIV drug- and sex-related risk behaviors.

Intervention Setting: A detention center.

Population: Of the 157 incarcerated, young, male drug users who participated in the study, 65% were African American, 33% were Hispanic, and 2% were white. The age of the participants ranged from 16 to 19 years.

Comparison Condition: The intervention was given to comparison participants at a later time.

Behavioral Findings: After release from jail, youth who participated in the intervention were significantly more likely to use condoms during vaginal, oral, and anal sex and had fewer high-risk sex partners than youth in the comparison condition.

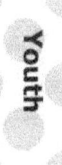

Youth

Drug Users

Description of Intervention: Intensive AIDS Education in Jail

The intervention was based on a problem-solving therapy model. It consisted of four 60-minute sessions focusing on health education issues relevant to male adolescent drug users, with emphasis on HIV/AIDS. The intervention was delivered at the New York City Department of Corrections Adolescent Reception and Detention Center on Rikers Island. Sessions used interactive methods and a small group format with 8 adolescents and one male counselor. Counselors were guided by a written curriculum.

Topics included general health knowledge, HIV and AIDS knowledge, factors associated with initiation and continuance of drug abuse, types of sexual behavior and HIV risk, the relationship of drug use and sexual behavior, and strategies to access services and drug abuse treatment in the community. Counselors adapted topics to the needs of the participants.

Counselors used techniques based on the problem-solving therapy model:

- *Problem orientation* - group members share and discuss facts and beliefs about HIV/AIDS
- *Problem definition and formulation* - members define specific high-risk attitudes and behaviors that must be modified to protect themselves and others against HIV/AIDS
- *Generation of alternative solutions* - members suggested and compiled possible courses of action for risky behaviors
- *Decision-making* - members critiqued and evaluated the alternative solutions
- *Solution implementation* - participants used role play and rehearsal techniques to practice alternative solutions.

The young men received $5 for each group session they attended.

Contact:

Stephen Magura
National Development and Research Institutes, Inc.
2 World Trade Center, 16th Floor
New York, NY 10048

Phone: 212–845–4521
Fax: 212–845–4698
E-mail: steve.magura@ndri.org

AIDS Education for Drug Abusers: Evaluation of Short-term Effectiveness

McCusker, J., Stoddard, A.M., Zapka, J.G., Morrison, C.S., et al. (1992).

American Journal of Public Health, 82 (4), 533 - 540

Intervention Goal(s): To determine the effects of small group Informational and Enhanced Education interventions on drug- and sex-related HIV risk behaviors.

Intervention Setting: Inpatient drug detoxification and rehabilitation center.

Description of Intervention: Informational and Enhanced AIDS Education

The interventions drew primarily from Social Cognitive Theory and Relapse Prevention Theory, and also included concepts from the Health Belief Model and Theory of Reasoned Action. The Informational Education intervention consisted of two 1-hour sessions. The Enhanced Education intervention was delivered in six 1-hour sessions. When the six sessions were completed, participants received a 30-minute individual health education consultation.

The Enhanced Education intervention focused on personal susceptibility, situation analysis and skills building. Participants engaged in group discussions and practiced skills they could use to reduce risk in various situations. Additional strategies were homework assignments, tension-release exercises, role-playing, trigger tapes, peer feedback, and needle cleaning and condom skills exercises. Emphasis was placed on experiential learning techniques for the purpose of enhancing participants' self-efficacy regarding their ability to initiate and maintain AIDS harm-reduction behaviors.

Population: Of the 567 adult drug users who participated in the study, 67% were men and 33% were women; 81% were white; and 70% were high school graduates.

Comparison Condition: Two one-hour sessions of essential HIV/AIDS information, using primarily didactic methods, including video, lecture, discussion, homework, and demonstration (but not practice) of condom use and cleaning of drug paraphernalia.

Behavioral Findings: After exit from the program, participants in both interventions reported significant reductions in drug- and sex-related risk behaviors compared with their baseline level of risk. For two behaviors, drug injection and cocaine use, the Enhanced Education intervention had significantly greater effects than the Informational Education intervention.

Contact:
Jane McCusker, MD, DrPH
Department of Clinical Epidemiology
and Community Studies
Room 2508, St. Mary's Hospital
3830 Lacombe Avenue
Montreal, Quebec, Canada H3T 1M5

Phone: 514–345–3511, ext. 5060
Fax: 514–734–2652
E-mail: janemc@ epid.lan.mcgill.ca

Condom Skills Education and Sexually Transmitted Disease Reinfection

Cohen, D., Dent, C., & MacKinnon, D. (1991).

Journal of Sex Research, 28 (1), 139 - 144

Intervention Goal(s): To determine the effects of a small group intervention on the incidence of sexually transmitted diseases (STDs).

Intervention Setting: Waiting room of an STD clinic.

Description of Intervention: Condom Skills Education

This intervention was based on the premise that familiarity with condoms and skills in using condoms properly are necessary for increasing future condom use. The intervention consisted of a brief condom skills education session led by a health educator who was an African-American woman. The intervention was delivered in a single 30-minute group session to people waiting for appointments in a Los Angeles STD clinic.

The session began with a 10- to 15-minute presentation in which the health educator emphasized 3 important points for effective condom use: condoms should be made of latex, condoms should have a reservoir tip or space left at the end, and condoms should be lubricated with a spermicide. The session included group discussion of how condoms should be used and a demonstration of how to put on a condom. The health educator referred to a poster that displayed a variety of condoms with their packaging. The presentation was followed by a 10- to 15-minute question-and-answer session.

Population: Of the 192 adults who participated in the study, 59% were male and 41% were female; 67% were African American, 15% were Hispanic, and 19% were of other racial/ethnic groups. The median age of the participants was 25 years, ranging from 15 to 61 years.

Comparison Condition: Usual services available in the STD clinic.

Behavioral/Health Findings: Men and women who participated in the intervention were significantly less likely to return to the STD clinic within the next 12 months with a new STD than those in the comparison condition.

Contact:

Deborah A. Cohen, MD, MPH
Department of Public Health and Preventive Medicine
1600 Canal Street
New Orleans, LA 70112

Phone: 504–680-9450
Fax: 504–680-9453
E-mail: dcohen@lsumc.edu

This study meets CDC's HIV/AIDS Prevention Research Synthesis project criteria for relevance and methodological rigor and also has the positive and significant behavioral/health findings required for the *Compendium.* Date added 1/99

1-7

Group Counseling at STD Clinics to Promote Use of Condoms

Cohen, D.A., MacKinnon, D.P., Dent, C., Mason, H., & Sullivan, E. (1992).

Public Health Reports, 107 (6), 727 - 731

Intervention Goal(s): To determine the effects of a small group intervention to promote safer sex and condom use.

Intervention Setting: Waiting room of an STD clinic.

Description of Intervention: Group Discussion Condom Promotion

This intervention used the social context of small groups to encourage change in norms, expectations, and social skills. The intervention was delivered in a single group session to people waiting for appointments in a Los Angeles STD clinic. A trained female African-American health educator led sessions for groups of 10-25 participants.

The intervention session began with a video, "Let's Do Something Different," depicting condom use as socially acceptable. After the video a health educator facilitated a group discussion on methods of preventing STDs and promoting condom use. This discussion included the reasons why people liked and disliked condoms. Role-playing gave the clinic patients an opportunity to practice condom negotiation, first with the health educator and then with another patient. Questions relating to medical aspects of STDs were referred to clinic nursing and medical personnel. All participants were offered 10 free condoms by clinic nurses.

Population: Of the 426 adults who participated in the study, 71% were men and 29% were women; 92% were African American. The average age of the participants was 28 years.

Comparison Condition: Usual services available in the STD clinic.

Behavioral/ Health Findings: Men who participated in the intervention had a significantly lower STD reinfection rate than men in the comparison condition. There was no evidence of change for women.

Contact:

Deborah A. Cohen, MD, MPH
Department of Public Health and Preventive Medicine
1600 Canal Street
New Orleans, LA 70112

Phone: 504–680-9450
Fax: 504–680-9453
E-mail: dcohen@lsumc.edu

This study meets CDC's HIV/AIDS Prevention Research Synthesis project criteria for relevance and methodological rigor and also has the positive and significant behavioral/health findings required for the *Compendium.* Date added 1/99

A Randomized Controlled Trial of an HIV Sexual Risk-reduction Intervention for Young African-American Women

DiClemente, R.J., & Wingood, GM. (1995).

Journal of the American Medical Association, 274 (16), 1271 - 1276

Intervention Goal(s): To determine the effects of a small group intervention to increase consistent condom use and prevent HIV infection.

Intervention Setting: Community center.[§]

Description of Intervention: Social Skills Training

Social Cognitive Theory and theories of gender and power were used as models to guide the development of this social skills intervention. The intervention consisted of five weekly 2-hour group sessions led by trained African-American peer educators in the Bayview-Hunter's Point community of San Francisco, California. Each session had a specific topic and planned activities for modeling and assessing skills.

Session 1: Gender and ethnic pride. The women discussed positive attributes of being an African-American woman.

Session 2: Personal responsibility for sexual decision making. The women watched an HIV prevention video and had discussion.

Session 3: Sexual assertiveness and communication training. Role-playing exercises were used to practice managing risky sexual situations.

Session 4: Condom use. The women concentrated on building skills and changing social norms for proper condom use.

Session 5: Cognitive coping skills. Participants developed skills such as sexual self-control.

Population: Among the 128 sexually active African-American women from an economically disadvantaged neighborhood who participated in the study, the average age was 23 years, ranging from 18-29 years.

Comparison Condition: The intervention was given to comparison participants at a later time.

Behavioral/Health Findings: Women who participated in the intervention were significantly more likely than women in the comparison condition to report consistent condom use with their partners, negotiating condom use, and not having sex when a condom was not available.

Contact:
Ralph DiClemente, PhD
Rollins School of Public Health
Emory University
1518 Clifton Road
Atlanta, GA 30022

Phone: 404–727–0237
Fax: 404–727–1369

§Information obtained from related reports or author.

Reducing Inner-city Women's AIDS Risk Activities: A Study of Single, Pregnant Women

Hobfoll, S.E., Jackson, A.P., Lavin, J., Britton, P.J., & Shepherd, J.B. (1994).

Health Psychology, 13 (5), 397 - 403

Intervention Goal(s): To determine the effects of a small group intervention to enhance AIDS knowledge, attitudes, and skills and, as a result, to influence behavior change.

Intervention Setting: Inner-city clinics for low-income women.

Population: Of the 206 single pregnant women who participated in the study, 57% were African American, 40% were white, and 3% were of other racial/ethnic groups. The average age of the participants was 21 years, ranging from 16 to 29 years. About one-third of the participants had not completed high school; 75% had income of less than $10,000 per year.

Description of Intervention: Reducing AIDS Risk Activities

The intervention was based on theories of social learning, conservation of resources (including coping strategies and support skills), and communal support.

Clinics were in a mid-sized Midwestern city. The intervention consisted of 4 sessions, 1½- to 2-hours each, for groups of 2 to 8 women. Trained group leaders were female psychologists and health educators whose ethnic backgrounds were similar to those of the participants.

Sessions featured videos using actors from the target population illustrating assertiveness, negotiation skills, planning skills, and specialized skills (e.g., cleaning drug works). Women discussed the videos and role-played risk scenarios. Participants created health plans.

Women learned negotiation skills and assertiveness skills. They developed a sense of mastery and positive expectations of success. The sessions also included an activity in which women imagined an unhealthy behavior and then imagined a healthy behavior. The final session addressed relapse prevention.

Incentives included cash, partial reimbursement for transportation and child care costs, and participation in a lottery for a color television.

Comparison Conditions: One was general health promotion, which included information, behavioral competency training, and social support that was not AIDS-specific, and the other was no intervention.

Behavioral Findings: Women who participated in the intervention increased their use of condoms with their partners more than women in the health promotion condition and significantly more than women who received no intervention.

Contact:
Stevan E. Hobfoll, PhD
Applied Psychology Center
Kent State University
P.O. Box 5190
Kent, OH 44242–0001

Phone: 330–672–2137
Fax: 330–672–3786
E-mail: shobfoll@kent.edu

This study meets CDC's HIV/AIDS Prevention Research Synthesis project criteria for relevance and methodological rigor and also has the positive and significant behavioral/health findings required for the *Compendium.* Date added 1/99

Efficacy of Risk-reduction Counseling to Prevent Human Immunodeficiency Virus and Sexually Transmitted Diseases: A Randomized Controlled Trial

Kamb, M.L., Fishbein, M., Douglas, J.M., Rhodes, F., et al. (1998).

Journal of the American Medical Association, 280 (13), 1161-1167

Intervention Goal(s): To determine the effects of enhanced and brief interactive counseling interventions to reduce high-risk behavior and to prevent new STDs.

Intervention Setting: Inner-city STD clinics.

Population: Of the 5,758 HIV-seronegative adults who participated in the study, 57% were male and 43% were female; 59% were African American, 19% were Hispanic, 16% were white, and 6% were of other racial/ethnic groups. Median age of the participants was 25 years and 24% were < 20 years; 54% were unemployed.

Description of Intervention: Project RESPECT§

The Enhanced and Brief Counseling interventions were based on the Theory of Reasoned Action and Social Cognitive Theory. Sessions were interactive and designed to change factors that could facilitate condom use, such as self-efficacy, attitudes, and perceived norms. The study was conducted in Baltimore, Denver, Long Beach, Newark, and San Francisco. Health department staff, trained to conduct HIV counseling, delivered the intervention.

The Enhanced Counseling intervention consisted of 4 sessions, a total of 200 minutes, and was completed in 3-4 weeks.

Session 1: Assessed personal risk, identified barriers to risk reduction, and negotiated a small risk-reduction step achievable in the next week.

Session 2: Explored condom use attitudes, discussed prior week's behavior change successes and barriers, and devised a strategy for taking a risk-reduction step before the next session.

Session 3: Received HIV test results, discussed prior week's behavioral goal and condom use barriers and facilitators, built condom use self-efficacy, and devised a strategy for taking another risk-reduction step.

Session 4: Explored social norms and support for condom use, discussed prior week's behavioral goal successes and barriers, and devised a long-term strategy for consistent condom use.

The Brief Counseling intervention consisted of 2 sessions, a total of 40 minutes, and was completed in 7-10 days. It was based on the HIV Prevention Counseling recommended by CDC for use with HIV testing since 1993.

Session 1: Identical to Session 1 above.

Session 2: Received HIV test results, discussed changes, support for changes made, and barriers and facilitators to change, and developed a long-term plan for risk reduction.

Incentives included cash for intervention sessions, follow-up visits, and STD exams.

Comparison Condition: Didactic messages typical of current care.

Behavioral Findings: Participants in both counseling interventions reported significantly higher condom use than participants in the comparison condition. Of the counseling participants, 30% fewer had new STDs than participants in the comparison condition. In the counseling interventions, benefits accrued equally to men and women, and STD reduction was higher among adolescents than older participants.

Contact:
Ken Hunt
Centers for Disease Control and Prevention
1600 Clifton Road, N.E. Mail Stop E-37
Atlanta, GA 30333

Phone: 404-639-2058
Fax: 404-639-1950
Email: khunt@cdc.gov

§Some information obtained from related reports or author.

This study meets CDC's HIV/AIDS Prevention Research Synthesis project criteria for relevance and methodological rigor and also has the positive and significant behavioral/health findings required for the *Compendium.* Date added 1/99

1-11

The Effects of HIV/AIDS Intervention Groups for High-risk Women in Urban Clinics

Kelly, J.A., Murphy, D.A., Washington, C.D., Wilson, T.S., et al., (1994).

American Journal of Public Health, 84(12), 1918 - 1922

Intervention Goal(s): To determine the effects of a small group intervention on high-risk behaviors.

Intervention Setting: Inner-city health clinic.

Population: Of the 197 women who were enrolled in the study, 87% were African American, 3% were Hispanic, 4% were American Indian, and 6% were white. The average age of participants was 29 years, and 97% of the whole group was unemployed. Average education level was some high school.

Description of Intervention: Cognitive-Behavioral Skills Training Group

The intervention incorporated cognitive-behavioral and risk-reduction skills training principles and peer support elements. It consisted of 4 weekly group sessions, 90 minutes each. There were 8 to 10 women in each group. The sessions were conducted in Milwaukee, Wisconsin by 2 female group leaders.

The sessions provided detailed information about HIV risk and focused on behaviors that increase risk, common misconceptions about AIDS, and steps to reduce the risk of contracting the disease. National and local HIV seroprevalence and epidemiology statistics were summarized to personalize risk situations for the women, including the possibility of encountering an infected partner.

Exercises emphasized cognitive-attitudinal areas, behavioral skills, and social factors. Participants role-played initiating discussion of concerns about AIDS and condom use with potential sex partners and resisting sexual pressure from a man whose risk history was unknown or with whom the woman did not want to have sex.

Skills-building was a critical component of this intervention. Condom demonstration and practice were provided to desensitize participants to condom use. Also, attention was directed toward recognizing, understanding, and managing one's personal triggers for high-risk behavior.

Comparison Condition: Family and child nutrition intervention.

Behavioral Findings: Women who participated in the intervention reported a significantly greater increase in condom use with their partners and a significantly greater decrease in their frequency of engaging in unprotected sex than women in the comparison condition.

Contact:
Jeffrey A. Kelly, PhD
Medical College of Wisconsin
2071 North Summit Avenue
Milwaukee, WI 53202

Phone: 414–456–7700
Fax: 414–287–4209
E-mail: jsherman@post.its.mcw.edu

A Community-level HIV Prevention Intervention for Inner-city Women: Results of the Women and Infants Demonstration Trial

Lauby, J.L., Smith, P.J., Stark, M., Person, B., & Adams, J. (2000).

American Journal of Public Health, 90 (2), 216 - 222

Intervention Goal(s): To determine the effects of a community-level intervention to increase condom use with main and other sex partners.

Intervention Setting: Street settings, community agencies, organizations, businesses, residential complexes, and other community settings.

Population: Interviews were conducted with 3,722 sexually active women of reproductive age. In this group of women, 73% were African-American, and the mean age was 25 years.

Comparison Condition: Usual HIV prevention programs available in matched communities.

Description of Intervention:
Women and Infants Demonstration Projects

This community-level intervention aimed to modify community norms, attitudes and behaviors concerning condom use among community women by providing models of successful risk-reduction strategies adopted by members of the target population. The intervention was based on the Transtheoretical Model of Behavior Change, which recognizes that change occurs in stages. The intervention was implemented over a 2-year period in four inner city communities in three metropolitan areas (Pittsburgh, West Philadelphia, and Portland).

The intervention included 3 components: a media campaign, outreach, and community mobilization. The media campaign included frequent distribution of flyers, brochures, posters, and newsletters that told "role model" stories based on the lives of women in the local community. These role model stories presented readable and realistic accounts of women in different degrees of readiness to use condoms (i.e., stage-based stories), how they had overcome barriers or had learned from experience about the need to use condoms, and how they had progressed to more consistent condom use.

Stage-based outreach was implemented by four trained full-time outreach specialists in each city. Outreach was usually one-on-one but was sometimes delivered to groups. The purpose of these interpersonal contacts was to provide tailored prevention messages, encourage and reinforce behavior change, and to distribute condoms and role model stories.

Community mobilization entailed the recruitment of peers to form a network of volunteers to provide HIV information, referrals, condoms, and the role model stories. Small businesses, neighborhood organizations, and agencies were also recruited to donate services or products and to function as sites for distributing role-model stories and displaying posters and other visual materials.

Behavioral/Health Findings:
Women in the intervention communities who were exposed to the intervention were more likely to have ever used condoms with main partners than women who were not exposed to the intervention in the comparison communities.

Contact:
Behavioral Intervention Research Branch
Division of HIV & AIDS Prevention
Centers for Disease Control and Prevention
1600 Clifton Road, MS E-37
Atlanta, GA 30333

Phone: 404-639-1900
Fax: 404-639-1950

This study meets CDC's HIV/AIDS Prevention Research Synthesis project criteria for relevance and methodological rigor and also has the positive and significant behavioral/health findings required for the *Compendium*. Date added 1/99

1-13

Reductions in STD Infections Subsequent to an STD Clinic Visit: Using Video-based Patient Education to Supplement Provider Interactions

O'Donnell, C.R., O'Donnell, L., San Doval, A., Duran, R., & Labes, K. (1998).

Sexually Transmitted Diseases, 25 (3), 161 - 168

Intervention Goal(s): To determine the effects of a small group intervention to reduce sexually transmitted disease (STD) infections subsequent to a clinic visit.

Intervention Setting: STD clinic.

Description of Intervention:
Video Opportunities for Innovative Condom Education and Safer Sex (VOICES/VOCES)

All participants received STD prevention information, individual counseling, free condoms, and a coupon for condoms as part of their clinic visit for diagnostic and treatment services.

The video-based intervention consisted of a 60-minute session in which participants viewed a 20-minute culturally sensitive video and engaged in a facilitated interactive group discussion. The intervention was delivered to small groups of 3 to 8 men in an STD clinic in the South Bronx, New York City. A trained STD counselor led the discussions.

One video, "Let's Do Something Different," was designed for African Americans and another, "Porque Sí," was developed for Hispanics. Both videos provided accurate risk information and corrected misinformation, portrayed positive attitudes about condom use, and modeled gender- and culturally-specific strategies for encouraging condom use. Interactive discussions following the videos aimed to reinforce the STD and HIV prevention messages. Participants addressed problems they had experienced when trying to use condoms and discussed strategies to increase condom use.

Participants were offered a selection of free condoms at the clinic and a coupon for free condoms at an area pharmacy.

Population: Of the 2004 adult males who participated in the study, 62% were African American and 38% were Hispanic. The average age of the participants was 30 years.

Comparison Condition: Usual services available in the STD clinic.

Behavioral Findings: Men who participated in the intervention had a significantly lower rate of new STD infection than men in the comparison condition.

Contact:
Lydia O'Donnell, EdD
Education Development Center, Inc.
55 Chapel Street
Newton, MA 02158

Phone: 617-969-7100, ext. 23
Fax: 617-969-3995
E-mail: lydiao@edc.org

This study meets CDC's HIV/AIDS Prevention Research Synthesis project criteria for relevance and methodological rigor and also has the positive and significant behavioral/health findings required for the *Compendium.* Date added 1/99

Reduction of High-risk Sexual Behavior among Heterosexuals Undergoing HIV Antibody Testing: A Randomized Control Trial

Wenger, N.S., Linn, L.S., Epstein, M., & Shapiro, M.F. (1991).

American Journal of Public Health, 81 (12), 1580 - 1585

Intervention Goal(s): To evaluate the effects of HIV education and testing on sexual risk behavior.

Intervention Setting: Urban STD clinic.

Description of Intervention: HIV Education, Testing, and Counseling

The intervention was offered to clients of an STD clinic in Los Angeles.

The intervention consisted of an educational component and an HIV blood test. The educational component included (a) a written pamphlet that explicitly discussed safer and unsafe sexual acts and explained condom use; (b) a 15-minute video that examined HIV-risk behavior and promoted condom use as well as discussing the risk with sex partners; and (c) a 10-minute, one-on-one counseling session with a physician.

The counseling session focused on assessing personal risk, discussing the elements of HIV testing, and answering any questions about HIV/AIDS or testing. [NOTE: See *Summary* for Kamb, et al. for current HIV testing and counseling protocols.]

After completing the educational module, intervention participants had blood drawn for an HIV test. Test results were revealed to intervention participants approximately 2 weeks after study entry and were accompanied by the same risk-reduction message as during the pretest counseling (for seronegative results) or in-depth counseling (for seropositive results).

Population: Of the 186 heterosexual adults who participated in the study, 67% were men and 33% were women; and 85% were African American; 84% had completed high school; and 43% were unemployed. The average age was 27 years.

Comparison Condition: HIV education only.

Behavioral Findings: Participants who received the HIV education and testing intervention reported significantly fewer occurrences of unprotected intercourse than did those in the comparison condition.

Contact:
Neil S. Wenger, MD
200 Medical Plaza
Suite 420
Los Angeles, CA 90095

Phone:	310–206–6232
Fax:	310–206–3551
E-mail:	nwenger@medicine.medsch.ucla.edu

The Mpowerment Project: A Community-level HIV Prevention Intervention for Young Gay Men

Kegeles, S.M., Hays, R.B., & Coates, T.J. (1996).

American Journal of Public Health, 86 (8), 1129 - 1136

Intervention Goal(s): To determine the effects of a community-level intervention to reduce HIV risk behaviors.

Intervention Setting: Mpowerment Center and other community venues where gay men congregated.

Population: Of the cohort of 300 young gay men who were evaluated after 8 months of study, 4% were African American, 7% were Asian or Pacific Islander, 6% were Hispanic, 81% were white, and 2% were of other racial/ethnic groups. The average age of the men was 23 years, and the median education level was some college.

Description of the Intervention: Mpowerment Project

This intervention was based on theories of peer influence and diffusion of innovations, which posit that people are most likely to adopt new behaviors when favorable evaluations of the behavior are conveyed to them by similar others whom they respect. The intervention was conducted over 8 months and attempted to reach all young gay men in a Eugene, Oregon community.

A Core Group of young gay men designed and ran the intervention with input from a Community Advisory Board composed of "elders" from the AIDS, public health, gay and lesbian, and university communities. This engendered a personal commitment to HIV prevention, a sense of ownership of the prevention activities, and a willingness to carry out the activities.

This multi-component intervention included 2 types of formal outreach, informal outreach, peer-led small groups, and a small ongoing publicity campaign. One type of formal outreach activity was directed at venues where young gay men congregated. Volunteers dressed in costumes and distributed safer-sex materials. Another type of formal outreach activity took place at the Mpowerment Center. It consisted of safer-sex promotional events embedded in a series of fun social activities. Informal outreach consisted of peer-initiated communications among friends about the need for safer sex. Small groups, called M-Groups, lasted about 3 hours and were designed to be fun and interactive. They served as entry into the project, addressed safer-sex concerns and skills, and motivated participants to invite their friends. The publicity campaign, which included articles and advertisements in gay newspapers and outreach materials, aimed to reinforce the norms for safer sex and spread awareness of the Mpowerment Project.

Comparison Condition: The intervention was given to comparison communities at a later time.

Behavioral Findings: Men who participated in the Mpowerment Project reduced their frequency of unprotected anal intercourse significantly more than the men in the comparison community.

Contact:
Ben Zovod
Center for AIDS Prevention Studies
University of California San Francisco
74 New Montgomery, Suite 600
San Francisco, CA 94105

Phone: 415–597–9306
Fax: 415–597–9213
E-mail: skegeles@psg.ucsf.edu

This study meets CDC's HIV/AIDS Prevention Research Synthesis project criteria for relevance and methodological rigor and also has the positive and significant behavioral/health findings required for the *Compendium*. Date added 1/99

Behavioral Intervention to Reduce AIDS Risk Activities

Kelly, J.A., St. Lawrence, J.S., Hood, H.V., & Brasfield, T.L. (1989)

Journal of Consulting and Clinical Psychology, 57 (1), 60 - 67

Intervention Goal(s): To determine the effects of a small group intervention to reduce the frequency of high-risk sexual practices and increase behavioral skills for refusing sexual coercions.

Intervention Setting: An office space associated with a medical center.[§]

Population: Of the 104 gay men who participated in the study, 13% were African American or Hispanic and 87% were white. The average age of the participants was 31 years; 45% had completed college.

Description of Intervention: Behavioral Self-management and Assertion Skills

The intervention consisted of 12 weekly group sessions, each about 75 to 90 minutes. Groups were led by 2 clinical psychologists and 2 project assistants.

Sessions 1-2: AIDS risk reduction. This component included information about AIDS, HIV infection, and HIV-transmission methods.

Sessions 3-5: Behavioral self-management. Participants examined past high-risk sexual activity and identified mood, setting, substance use, and other factors associated with the risk taking. Leaders presented strategies to reduce risk.

Sessions 6-8: Assertion skills training. Three scenarios were used: (a) initiating discussion about one's commitment to low-risk behavior with a potential sex partner; (b) refusing pressures to engage in high-risk behavior; and (c) declining an immediate sexual proposition from a person one wanted to get to know socially.

Sessions 9-11: Relationship skills and social support development. This component addressed strategies for problem solving in relationships and for maintaining low-risk sexual practices, even in committed relationships.

Session 12: Risk-reduction review and identification of useful strategies. This session allowed each participant to address the changes he had made and the strategies he had used.

The intervention used group process, lecture, and role-playing methods to deliver information and develop skills.

Comparison Condition: The intervention was given to comparison participants at a later time

Behavioral Findings: Gay men who participated in the intervention reduced their frequency of unprotected anal intercourse and increased their use of condoms significantly more than the men in the comparison condition.

Contact:
Jeffrey A. Kelly, PhD
Medical College of Wisconsin
2071 North Summit Avenue
Milwaukee, WI 53202

Phone: 414–456–7700
Fax: 414–287–4209
E-mail: jsherman@post.its.mcw.edu

§Information obtained from related reports or author.

This study meets CDC's HIV/AIDS Prevention Research Synthesis project criteria for relevance and methodological rigor and also has the positive and significant behavioral/health findings required for the *Compendium.* Date added 1/99

1-17

HIV Risk Behavior Reduction Following Intervention with Key Opinion Leaders of Population: An Experimental Analysis

Kelly, J.A., St. Lawrence, J.S., Diaz, Y.E. Stevenson, L.Y., et al. (1991).

American Journal of Public Health, 81 (2), 168 - 171

Intervention Goal(s): To determine the effects of a community-level intervention to reduce high-risk behaviors.

Intervention Setting: Gay bars.[§]

Population: Of the 659 gay men who completed anonymous baseline surveys, 14% were African American or Hispanic, and 86% were white. Average age was 29 years.

Comparison Condition: The intervention was given to comparison participants at a later time.

Description of Intervention: Popular Opinion Leader (POL)

This intervention was based on theories of peer influence, behavioral standards and social norms, and diffusion of innovations. Bartenders at gay clubs in Biloxi, Mississippi, Monroe, Louisiana, and Hattiesburg, Mississippi were enlisted to nominate opinion leaders, i.e., persons who were popular with others. The intervention was delivered in two parts:

Part I. Popular opinion leaders received four sessions, 90 minutes each[§], of HIV education and communication strategies. A male and a female co-facilitator conducted each session.

Session 1: Epidemiology of HIV, risk and protective behaviors, and misconceptions.

Session 2: Characteristics of effective health promotion messages. Facilitators described ways to sensitize others to the threat of AIDS, stressed that behavior change can prevent AIDS, used self as example, and personally endorsed the benefits of change.

Session 3: Conversational examples of effective health promotion messages. Facilitators modeled conversations and opinion leader participants role-played similar conversations.

Session 4: Real-life conversations and problem solving. Participants reported outcomes of actual conversations (see Part II). Facilitators helped them plan for additional peer conversations.

Part II. Each opinion leader agreed to have at least 14 conversations with peers in the bars about AIDS risk reduction. Opinion leaders wore buttons with a logo that promoted the project and matched posters located in the bars. Buttons were ambiguous and served to trigger conversations.

Behavioral Findings: Men from the community that received the intervention reported a significantly greater reduction in unprotected anal intercourse than the men from the comparison communities.

Contact:
Jeffrey A. Kelly, PhD
Medical College of Wisconsin
2071 North Summit Avenue
Milwaukee, WI 53202

Phone:	414–456–7700
Fax:	414–287–4209
E-mail:	jsherman@post.its.mcw.edu

AIDS Prevention in Homosexual and Bisexual Men: Results of a Randomized Trial Evaluating Two Risk Reduction Interventions

Valdiserri, R.O., Lyter, D.W., Leviton, L.C., Callahan, C.M., et al. (1989).

AIDS, 3 (1), 21 - 26

Intervention Goal(s): To determine the effects of an educational intervention program that included skills training in addition to a small group lecture on sexual risk and protective behaviors.

Intervention Setting: The office of a community-based organization.

Population: Of the 584 gay and bisexual men who participated in the study, 2% were African American, less than 1% were Hispanic, less than 1% were Asian, and 95% were white. The average age was 33 years, ranging from 19 to 73 years, and 33% of the participants had a college degree.

Comparison Condition: Small group lecture.

Behavioral Findings: Men who participated in the small group lecture plus skills training educational intervention showed a significant increase in condom use for insertive anal intercourse compared to those in the comparison condition.

Contact:
Ronald O. Valdiserri, MD, MPH
Centers for Disease Control and Prevention
1600 Clifton Road
Mail Stop E–07
Atlanta, GA 30333

Phone: 404–639–8002
Fax: 404–639–8600
E-mail: ROV1@cdc.gov

Description of Intervention: Small Group Lecture Plus Skills Training

The intervention consisted of a lecture and a skills training session delivered in a 2-session small group format in a community-based organization in Pittsburgh, Pennsylvania. The 60- to 90-minute lecture component, led by a gay health educator, reviewed HIV transmission and the clinical outcomes of HIV infection, the risks of specific sexual practices, the importance of risk reduction through safer-sex practices, correct condom use, and interpretation of HIV antibody tests.

The 140-minute skills-training session was led by a psychotherapist from a community organization that provides counseling services to sexual minorities. The skills-training session included role-playing, psychodrama, and group process to promote the social acceptability of safer sex; strategies to reduce sexual risk behavior; and group discussion on sexuality and relationships among gay men.

Men Who Have Sex With Men

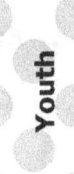

Youth

Reductions in HIV Risk-associated Sexual Behaviors among Black Male Adolescents: Effects of an AIDS Prevention Intervention

Jemmott, J.B., Jemmott, L.S., & Fong, G.T. (1992).

American Journal of Public Health, 82 (3), 372 - 377

Intervention Goal(s): To determine the effects of a small group intervention to reduce HIV risk behaviors and increase condom use.

Intervention Setting: A local school on a Saturday.

Population: Of the 157 African-American male adolescents who participated in the study, the average age of participants was 15 years; almost all (97%) were enrolled in school.

Comparison Condition: Career planning and opportunities, structurally similar to the intervention.

Behavioral Findings: Adolescents who participated in the intervention reported more frequent use of condoms and fewer sex partners than adolescents in the comparison condition.

Description of Intervention: Be Proud! Be Responsible!

The intervention consisted of one 5-hour session held on a Saturday morning in a local school in Philadelphia, Pennsylvania. The session was led by African-American men and women with backgrounds in human sexuality education, nursing, social work, and small group facilitation. The leaders received 6 hours of training for this intervention. The intervention included information about risks associated with injection drug use and specific sexual activities. The intervention used videos, games, exercises, and other culturally and developmentally appropriate materials to reinforce learning and to encourage active participation.

For example, one video was narrated by an African-American woman and had a multi-ethnic cast.

In another activity, "AIDS Basketball," participants formed into teams to earn points for correctly answering factual questions on AIDS. In the exercise, "Uncle Bill's Advice Column," pairs of adolescents wrote a response to a letter to Uncle Bill about AIDS or risky behavior and then read it to the rest of the group for discussion.

A condom exercise focused on the correct use of condoms. The participants also engaged in role-playing situations depicting potential problems in trying to implement safer sex practices, including abstinence.

Contact:
John B. Jemmott III, PhD
University of Pennsylvania
Center for Health Behavior &
Communication Research
3535 Market Street, Suite 520
Philadelphia, PA 19104-3309

Phone: 215-573-9366
Fax: 215-573-9303
E-mail: jjemmott@asc.upenn.edu

This study meets CDC's HIV/AIDS Prevention Research Synthesis project criteria for relevance and methodological rigor and also has the positive and significant behavioral/health findings required for the *Compendium*. Date added 1/99

Reducing the Risk: Impact of a New Curriculum on Sexual Risk-taking

Kirby, D., Barth, R.P., Leland, N., & Fetro, J.V. (1991).

Family Planning Perspectives, 23 (6), 253 - 263

Intervention Goal(s): To determine the effects of a classroom intervention to postpone initiation of sexual intercourse and, among those sexually experienced, to reduce unprotected sex.

Intervention Setting: High school classrooms.

Population: Of the 758 students who participated in the study, 47% were male and 53% were female; 2% were African American, 2% were American Indian, 9% were Asian, 20% were Hispanic, 62% were white, and 5% were of other racial/ethnic groups. The average age was 15 years, and about 37% of the participants were sexually experienced prior to the study.

Description of Intervention: Reducing the Risk

The intervention was based on social learning, social inoculation, and cognitive behavioral theories. The intervention was carried out in 13 high schools in California. Health education classes offered the 15-session intervention as part of the 10th grade comprehensive health curriculum. Teachers who volunteered to implement the intervention curriculum attended a 3-day training session.

The curriculum included instruction on developing social skills to reduce sexual risk-taking behavior and used role play as a means of practicing and modeling those skills. Numerous activities supported the norm that students should avoid unprotected intercourse, either by not having sex or by using contraceptives. Students repeatedly role played situations where they recognized various forms of social pressure to have sex, examined the "lines" that young people use to obtain sex, were motivated to resist these pressures, and practiced effective strategies and skills to refrain from sex or unprotected sex. Over the 15 weeks, role plays were less scripted and more oriented to developing student's confidence in their ability to resist pressure. The curriculum also emphasized decision making and assertive communication skills, encouraged students to go to stores and clinics to obtain relevant health information, and required students to ask their parents about their views on abstinence and birth control.

Comparison Condition: Usual sexuality instruction available in the school.

Behavioral Findings: Students receiving the intervention were significantly less likely to initiate sexual intercourse than those in the comparison condition; intervention students who were already sexually experienced were significantly less likely to engage in unprotected intercourse than sexually active students in the comparison condition.

Contact:
Nancy Shanfeld, PhD
ETR Associates
P.O. Box 1830
Santa Cruz, CA 95061

Phone: 408–438–4060
Fax: 408–438–4618

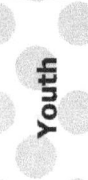

Preventing HIV Infection Among Adolescents: Evaluation of a School-based Education Program

Main, D.S., Iverson, D.C., McGloin, J., Banspach, S.W., et al. (1994).

Preventive Medicine, 23 (4), 409 - 417

Intervention Goal(s): To determine the effects of a classroom intervention to postpone the initiation of sexual intercourse and to reduce the number of students engaging in unsafe sex and drug-using behaviors.

Description of Intervention: Get Real about AIDS© 1992

This intervention was primarily based on Social Cognitive Theory and the Theory of Reasoned Action. The intervention was implemented in 10 schools in 6 Colorado school districts. The intervention consisted of a 15-session skills-based curriculum, based in part on the program Get Real About AIDS© 1992. Most of the intervention teachers taught health; some taught science, physical education, and study skills. Teachers attended a 5-day (40 hours) training program designed to enhance relevant skills and fidelity of the implementation to the written curriculum.

The curriculum covered the following topics: HIV functional knowledge (that is, knowledge that can be used to reduce risk), teen vulnerability to HIV, normative determinants of risky behavior, condom use, and skills designed to help students recognize, manage, avoid, or leave risky situations.

Intervention Setting: High school classrooms.

Population: Of the 2,015 students who participated in the study, 51% were male and 49% were female; 6% were African American, 3% were Asian, 21% were Hispanic, 65% were white, and 5% were of other racial/ethnic groups. The average age of the students was 15 years; 60% were in the 9th grade; 44% were sexually experienced prior to the study.

Comparison Condition: Usual program, which was no HIV education or minimal HIV education, as determined by the school districts.

Behavioral Findings: Students who participated in the intervention reported fewer sex partners and greater frequency of condom use than students in the comparison schools.

Contact:
Deborah S. Main, PhD
Department of Family Medicine
1180 Clermont Street
Denver, Colorado 80220

Phone: 303–315–9700
Fax: 303–315–9747
E-mail: debbi.main@uchsc.edu

Reductions in HIV Risk among Runaway Youths

Rotheram-Borus, M., Van Rossem, R., Gwadz, M., Koopman, C., & Lee, M. (1997)

University of California, Department of Psychiatry, Division of Social and Community Psychiatry, Los Angeles, CA

Intervention Goal(s): To determine the effects of a small group intervention to reduce HIV-related sexual and drug-related risk behaviors.

Intervention Setting: Shelters for runaway adolescents.

Population: Of the 312 runaway and homeless youths who enrolled in the study, 51% were male and 49% were female; 57% were African American, 22% were Hispanic, 16% were white or of other racial/ethnic groups, and race/ethnicity was unknown for 5%. The average age of the youths was 16 years.

Comparison Condition: Usual services available in the runaway shelters.

Behavioral Findings: Adolescents who participated in the intervention reduced both the number of unprotected sexual acts and their substance use significantly more than adolescents in the comparison shelters.

Contact:
Mary Jane Rotheram-Borus, PhD
Department of Psychiatry
University of California Los Angeles
10920 Wilshire Blvd, Suite 350
Los Angeles, CA 90024

Phone: 310–794–8278
Fax: 310–794–8297
E-mail: rotheram@ucla.edu

Description of Intervention: StreetSmart
This intervention was based on Social Learning Theory, using small groups (a) as practice and role-play opportunities, (b) to mobilize and reinforce positive behaviors, and (c) to maintain support networks. The intervention consisted of 10 group sessions on a rotating basis, 3 times per week, repeated every 4 to 6 weeks, and one individual counseling session. Sessions were led by trained counselors in shelters for runaway youth in the New York City area. The intervention had four primary components:

1. HIV-related knowledge. Activities included video and art workshops where youth developed soap opera dramatizations, public service announcements, commercials, and raps about HIV prevention, and they reviewed and discussed commercial HIV/AIDS prevention videos.

2. Social skills. Training on assertiveness and coping skills, including use of a "feeling thermometer," were employed to develop skills for use in HIV-risk situations.

3. Access to resources. Participants visited a community based comprehensive health and mental health center.

4. Personalized beliefs, attitudes and norms. Participants had a private counseling session during which they could assess individual barriers to practicing safer sex and discuss their own attitudes and behavior patterns. Dysfunctional attitudes and behavior patterns were targeted.

Incentives included food and $1 for carrying condoms and arriving to the program on time.

A Randomized, Controlled Effectiveness Trial of an AIDS Prevention Program for Low-income African-American Youths

Stanton, B.F., Li, X., Ricardo, I., Galbraith, J., Feigelman, S., & Kaljee, L. (1996).

Archives of Pediatrics and Adolescent Medicine, 150 (4), 363 - 372

Intervention Goal(s): To determine the effects of a peer network decision-making intervention to increase condom use among sexually active youth.

Intervention Setting: Recreation centers associated with public housing developments; rural campsite setting.

Population: Of the 383 African-American youths who participated in the study, 56% were male and 44% were female. The average age was 11 years, ranging from 9 to 15 years; 36% were sexually experienced prior to the study.

Description of Intervention: Focus on Kids

The intervention, developed through ethnographic research, targeted pre- and early-adolescents in their existing friendship groups. Being in such a group was a requirement of enrollment. AIDS prevention education was based on a social cognitive model, Protection Motivation Theory (PMT), that uses cost and reward constructs to explain how intentions are formed to respond to threats in either adaptive or maladaptive ways.

The intervention consisted of 8 sessions: seven 1½-hour weekly meetings at local recreational centers and one day-long session at a rural campsite. The intervention was delivered in a large Eastern city to peer groups that consisted of 3 to 10 same-gender friends within 3 years of age of each other. The sessions were led by a pair of interventionists, at least one of whom was gender matched to the group. Most of the interventionists were African-American men and women recruited from the community.

Each session focused on one or more PMT concepts and also reviewed concepts from the prior session. Beginning in the first session and integrated throughout, a family genogram was used to illustrate the application of concepts to real-life situations.

Sessions emphasized values clarification and goal setting; presented facts regarding AIDS, STDs, contraception, and human development; and provided condoms. Multiple delivery formats were used to address individual variability in receptivity to media, e.g., videos, games, role-playing, acting, storytelling, and arts and crafts.

In the seventh session, participants developed community projects with specific target audiences and intervention messages. The eighth session included a presentation of the projects and concluded with a "graduation" ceremony.

Comparison Condition: Individual youth attended weekly sessions, which included a movie with AIDS facts, discussion, and access to condoms.

Behavioral Findings: Sexually active youth who participated in the intervention reported significantly greater condom use than sexually active youth in the comparison condition.

Contact:
Bonita Stanton, MD
Department of Pediatrics
University of Maryland at Baltimore
700 West Lombard Street
Baltimore, MD 21201

Phone: 410–706–5289
Fax: 410–706–0653
E-mail: bstanton@umabnet.ab.umd.edu

Cognitive-Behavioral Intervention To Reduce African-American Adolescents' Risk for HIV Infection

St. Lawrence, J.S., Brasfield, T.L., Jefferson, K.W., Alleyne, E., O'Bannon, R.E., & Shirley, A. (1995).

Journal of Consulting and Clinical Psychology, 63 (2), 221 - 237

Intervention Goal(s): To determine the effects a small group intervention.

Intervention Setting: A public health clinic serving low-income families.[§]

Population: Of the 246 inner city African-American youths who enrolled in the study, 28% were male and 72% were female. The average age was 15 years; the average school grade was 10; and 36% were sexually experienced prior to the study.

Comparison Condition: Received Session 1 only.

Behavioral Findings: Youths who participated in the intervention reported significantly greater condom use and significantly lower frequency of unprotected intercourse than youths in the comparison condition. Abstinent youth who participated in the intervention significantly delayed sexual onset to a greater extent than abstinent youth in the comparison condition.

Description of Intervention: Becoming A Responsible Teen (BART)

This intervention is based on social learning theory and stresses attention to participants' informational needs, motivational influences, and behavior (IMB), from the IMB risk-reduction model. The intervention consisted of 8 weekly educational and behavior skills sessions of 90 to 120 minutes each. Two co-facilitators, a male and a female, led the sessions in a small group format. The intervention was conducted in a comprehensive health center that serves predominantly low-income minority clients in a Mississippi city of 400,000 residents.

Session 1: AIDS education. HIV/AIDS information, presented in the context of local HIV/AIDS demographics, was interspersed with games, group discussion, and other activities.

Session 2: Sexual decisions and values. Group discussion about sexual decisions and pressures was followed by a video for African-American youths, *Seriously Fresh*, and video discussion.

Session 3: Technical competency skills. Discussion of statewide adolescent sexual activity levels was followed by condom use demonstrations, small group practice, and cognitive restructuring of unhelpful beliefs about self-protection and condom use.

Session 4-6: Social competency skills. Communication skills and assertiveness were taught in 3 contexts: a) initiating discussion about condoms in advance with a sex partner, b) refusing pressure to engage in unprotected sex, and c) sharing HIV-risk information with peers. Leaders demonstrated these skills, followed by participant role play.

Session 7: Cognitive competency skills. Local HIV-seropositive youths, the "Rap Team," discussed how HIV had affected their lives. Behavioral self-management and problem-solving strategies, especially those used successfully in the past, were the focus of sessions 7 and 8.

Session 8: Social support and empowerment. Participants shared what each felt was most helpful in BART and the personal changes each had made in response to participating in BART. The impact the group could have by educating friends and families was illustrated and the importance of supportive friendship networks was stressed.

Incentives included $5 an hour for participation, a project T-shirt for attending all sessions, and a personalized certificate of completion.

§Information obtained from related reports or author.

Contact:
Janet S. St. Lawrence, PhD
Centers for Disease Control and Prevention
1600 Clifton Road, Mail Stop E–44
Atlanta, GA 30333

Phone: 404–639–8298
Fax: 404–639–8622
E-mail: nzs4@cdc.gov

Section 2
Tables

Table 1.

POPULATION CHARACTERISTICS
Gender, Race/Ethnicity, and Age

INTERVENTION CHARACTERISTICS
Setting, Level, and Duration

Citation	Target				Gender %		Race/Ethnicity %						Age (Yrs.)		Setting	Level			Duration	
	DU	HA	MSM	Y	M	F	A-A	API	H	AI	W	O	Mean	Range		Ind	Grp	Com	#Sessions	Total time
ACDP '99	■	■			45	55	54		19		22	5		11-87	Community	✓		✓	Continuous - 3 yrs	
Cohen '91					59	41	67		15			19	25*	15-61	Health Care		✓		1	≥10 min
Cohen '92					71	29	92#						29		Health Care		✓		1	NR
Des Jarlais '92			■		70	30	26		23		51		27	16-48	Storefront§	✓	✓		6	≥4-6 hr
DiClemente '95						100	100						23	18-29	Community§		✓		5	10 hr
El-Bassel '92						100	36§		64§				35		Health Care§		✓		5	5 hrs§
Hobfoll '94						100	57				40	3	21	16-29	Health Care§		✓		4	6-8 hr
Jemmott '92					100		100						15		Educational		✓		1	5 hr
Kamb '98					57	43	59		19		16	6	25*		Health Care	✓			Enhan: 4 / Brief: 2	3hr 20min / 40 min
Kegeles '96			■		100		4	7	6		81	2	23		HIV/AIDS Venue Public Access Commercial	✓	✓	✓	Continuous - 8 mos	
Kelly '89			■		100		13◊		◊		87		31		Med. Office§	✓			12	15-18 hr
Kelly '91			■		100		14◊		◊		86		29		Gay Bars§	✓§	✓§	✓§	NA	NA
Kelly '94						100	87		3	4	6		29		Health Care		✓		5	> 6 hr
Kirby '91					47	53	2	9	20	2	62	5	15		Educational		✓	✓	15 classes	~15 hr
Lauby '00						100	73#						25		CBE Public Access Commercial		✓	✓	Continuous - 2 yrs	
Magura '94					100		65		33		2			16-19	Correctional Facility	✓	✓		4	4 hr
Main '94					51	49	6	3	21		65	5	15		Educational		✓		15 classes	~15 hr
McCusker '92					67	33					81#		NR		Health Care	✓	✓		8	> 6.5 hr
O'Donnell '98					100		62		38				30		Health Care	✓	✓		1§	1 hr§
Rotheram-Borus '97					51	49	57		22		16†	5‡	16		CBE	✓	✓		10	NR
Stanton '96				■	56	44	100						11	9-15	CBE Public Access		✓		7 + 1 retreat	10.5 hr + "all day"
St. Lawrence '95				■	28	72	100	1	1				15		HealthCare§		✓		8	12-16 hr
Valdiserri '89					100		2	1	1		95		33	19-73	NR	✓			1	2hr 20min
Wenger '91					67	33	85#						27		Health Care	✓			2	>25 min

DU = Drug Users; HA = Heterosexual Adults; MSM = Men who have Sex with Men; Y = Youth; NR = Not Reported; Ind = Individual; Grp = Group; Com = Community
CBE = Community-Based Establishment (non-commercial, community service site, e.g., a shelter); Enhan = Enhanced; A-A = African American; API = Asian / Pacific Islander; H = Hispanic; AI = American Indian; W = White; O = Other than specified †Combined white and other than specified; ◊A-A and H combined; ‡race/ethnicity reported as unknown; # race/ethnicity not reported on 100% of the study population; *median age given instead of mean age; §Data obtained from related reports or author

CDC's HIV/AIDS Prevention Research Synthesis Project, 404-639-1900, November 1999

Table 2.
Interventions with CDC Support for Materials Production, Technical Assistance, and Training

Table 2 lists the interventions that receive CDC support through either Replicating Effective Programs (REP)[1*] or the Prevention Counseling Course Series[2] in CDC's Division of HIV/AIDS Prevention or Research to Classroom: Programs That Work (PTW)[3] in CDC's Division of Adolescent and School Health. Since some of the REP and PTW studies were recently funded, some materials are not yet available.[**]

Author of Study & Materials Developer	Intervention Name	Target Population	Study Funding Source	Materials Available*
ADCP, 1999 Materials by Corby – Community PROMISE	AIDS Community Demo. Proj.	All Categories	CDC	In Progress[1]
Kamb, 1998	Project RESPECT	Heterosexual Adults	CDC	Yes[2]
Lauby 2000 Materials by Adams – Pittsburg site only Real AIDS Prevention Project (RAPP)	WIDP	Heterosexual Adults	CDC	Yes[1]
O'Donnell, 1998	VOICES/VOCES	Heterosexual Adults	CDC	Yes[1]
Kegeles, 1996	Mpowerment Project	Men Who Have Sex With Men	NIMH	Yes[1]
Kelly, 1991	Popular Opinion Leader (POL)	Men Who Have Sex With Men	NIMH	Yes[1]
Jemmott, 1992	Be Proud! Be Responsible!	Youth	NIMH	Yes[3]
Kirby, 1991	Reducing the Risk	Youth	Private foundations, NIH	Yes[3]
Main, 1994	Get Real about AIDS © 1992	Youth	CDC	Yes[3]
Rotheram-Borus, 1997	StreetSmart	Youth	NIMH	Yes[1]
Stanton, 1996	Focus on Kids	Youth	NIMH	Yes[3]
St. Lawrence, 1995	Becoming a Responsible Teen (BART)	Youth	NIMH	Yes[3]

*In 1996 CDC's Division of HIV/AIDS Prevention - Intervention Research and Support initiated Replicating Effective Programs (REP) to support the development and dissemination of materials for interventions with evidence of effectiveness. To be eligible, interventions must have met PRS and *Compendium* criteria (see Appendix A). In the first years, REP support was given to the developers of completed studies that met the specified criteria, regardless of source of the original research funding. In future years, when CDC funded studies show positive behavioral/health results, CDC will continue to support and seek to provide additional funds for development and dissemination. We encourage other funding agencies to do the same.

**Five other studies listed in the Compendium (Cohen et al. '92, DesJarlais '92, DiClemente & Wingood '95, McCusker et al. '92, and Valdiserri et al. '89) are reported to have intervention packages available commercially: J.J. Card, T. Benner, J.P. Shields, and N. Feinstein. The HIV/AIDS Prevention Program Archive (HAPPA): A Collection of Promising Prevention Programs in a Box. *AIDS Education and Prevention*, 13(1), 1-28, 2001.

Section 3
Intervention Checklist

Intervention Checklist:
Elements of Successful Programs
A Tool for Assessment of Local HIV/AIDS Interventions

Background

The *Compendium* provides ready access to many interventions with known effectiveness, however, program planners, managers, or prevention service providers may be using an existing intervention that has its own advantages. For instance, it was developed locally and there is consensus in the community about its value. The *Intervention Checklist* was developed as a tool to help with assessment of these existing interventions. *Checklist* items were derived primarily from the common characteristics of successful programs in the Reputationally Strong Programs Project (RSP), funded by CDC. Public and private AIDS organizations and CDC Project Officers nominated HIV prevention programs that were viewed as "strong" because of their innovation, organizational characteristics, field experience, and contributions to our understanding of intervention. Eligible programs had to be located in the U.S., be locally based, be currently operational, have a strong reputation for showing promise for preventing HIV, and could not have been formally evaluated

How to Use This Tool

One may want to use the *Checklist* to fine-tune a strong program, or to consider new ideas for program implementation or organizational planning. It may be helpful simply as a programmatic inventory. This tool could be used in a regular staff or planning group meeting or an annual program review to help measure progress.

Instructions:

1. Consider each of the four sections and each item within the sections. It may be useful to record examples from your local intervention onto the form in the space provided (if needed, use bottom, back of page, etc.) Also, you may want to add items.
2. Working individually or in a group, complete the *Checklist*. Rate each item High, Medium, or Low. For instance, for the first Intervention item, a clearly defined audience, a "high" rating would mean that the audience is very clearly defined, i.e., with enough precision (e.g., ethnically/culturally, by risk behavior, gender, or other characteristics) for optimal planning, tailoring of materials to that audience, and targeted recruitment.
3. Review your responses. Consider each section separately. For example, are there one or two items in the Implementation section that need attention?
4. How do you/your group assess the current intervention overall? Is it satisfactory or can it be strengthened? If you want to improve the activity, who would develop an action plan for that? What accomplishment would address your current concerns? How feasible is that? What technical assistance might be helpful? What time lines would you anticipate? What resources would be needed?

[1] **References**

Holtgrave, D.R., et al. (1995). An overview of the effectiveness and efficiency of HIV prevention programs. *Public Health Reports*, 110 (2), 134-146.

Janz, N.K., et al. (1996). Evaluation of 37 AIDS prevention projects: successful approaches and barriers to program effectiveness. *Health Education Quarterly*, 23 (1), 80-97.

Mezoff, J., Seals, B., Sogolow, E., Komescher, R., Wooden, G, Bye, L., Tijugum, B. (1998). Reputationally Strong HIV Prevention Programs: Organizational Characteristics. Poster presentation, 12th World AIDS Conference, Geneva.

Kirby, D. (1995). A review of educational programs designed to reduce sexual risk-taking behaviors among school-aged youth in the United States. In *The Effectiveness of AIDS Prevention Efforts, HIV Prevention: State-of-the-Science*, commissioned by the Office of Technology Assessment, compiled and produced by the American Psychological Association Office on AIDS, Washington, D.C.

CDC's HIV/AIDS Prevention Research Synthesis Project, 404-639-1900, November 1999

A. Intervention Items	Examples from Effective Interventions	Examples from Local Interventions (Write In)	Rating (Circle One)
1. The intervention has a clearly defined audience	STD patients who are at risk based on current STD infection Runaway youth living in shelters who are at risk through survival sex		High Medium Low
2. The intervention has clearly defined goals and objectives	To change risky sexual norms and behaviors in the gay community through personal endorsement of safer sex by key opinion leaders To reduce risk for HIV/STD and unintended pregnancy among young women by increasing condom use		High Medium Low
3. The intervention is based on sound behavioral and social science theory	Diffusion theory guides plan for key opinion leaders to speak with certain number of people (representing proportion of the at-risk population) Stages of change model calls for tailoring the role model stories used in the intervention to level of readiness for risk reduction in the community		High Medium Low
4. The intervention is focused on reducing specific risk behaviors	Reduce unprotected anal sex among men who have sex with men Reduce "never using" condoms with steady and casual sex partners		High Medium Low
5. The intervention provides opportunities to practice relevant skills	Role play condom negotiation with steady sex partner Exercises for trying out personal coping strategies		High Medium Low

B. Implementation Items	Examples from Effective Interventions	Examples from Local Interventions (Write In)	Rating (Circle One)
1. There is a realistic schedule for implementation	Six months of preparation and coordination is needed before starting an intervention in a large health care organization Two years of implementation are required for community level change		High Medium Low
2. Staff are adequately trained for sensitivity to the target population	Staff receive training on responding to disclosures of domestic violence Staff attend three, 1 hour sessions on the target population's culture, risk factors, and barriers to accessing service		High Medium Low
3. Staff are adequately trained to deliver the core elements of the intervention	Peer volunteers receive 32 hours of interactive training on the intervention's goals, objectives, core elements, and delivery methods Staff read intervention manuals, view training videos, role play intervention delivery, and have "booster" training one month after starting the intervention		High Medium Low
4. Core elements of the intervention are clearly defined and maintained in the delivery	Health educators use an intervention manual that labels the core elements Supervisor observes intervention performance at least once a month and provides feedback on delivery of the core elements		High Medium Low
5. Staff uses a variety of teaching methods, strategies, and modalities to convey information, personalize the training, and repeat essential HIV prevention messages	Lecture, discussion, group art and music projects, stress coping exercises, and individual counseling Staff use of culturally specific video soap opera as a springboard for problem solving client's barriers to condom negotiation; condom information is repeated in large-scale poster format		High Medium Low

C. Organization Items	Examples from Effective Interventions	Examples from Local Interventions (Write In)	Rating (Circle One)
1. There is administrative support for the intervention at the highest levels	State health department commits to delivering the intervention in all STD, HIV, and family planning clinics holding state contracts Local public housing authority provides on site office space for intervention activities		High Medium Low
2. There are sufficient resources for the current implementation	Existing facility incorporates intervention into its continuum of care by replacing didactic information delivery with an information and skills-building intervention Suitable space for the activities is located and rent is paid		High Medium Low
3. There are sufficient resources for sustainability	Redefinition of duties makes intervention delivery part of staff job description Intervention is not tied to grant funding but is part of agency's overall budget		High Medium Low
4. Decision-makers are flexible and open to program changes	"Ownership" of project is shared with target population volunteers who select new venues for delivery Non-agency staff are permitted to deliver intervention to agency clients on-site		High Medium Low
5. HIV/AIDS intervention is embedded in a broader context that is relevant to the target population	Runaway youth receive shelter, medical care, mental health counseling, and service referrals in addition to HIV prevention intervention Inner city women receive HIV/AIDS intervention woven into the context of women's health, pregnancy planning, and caring for one's family		High Medium Low

D. Consumer/ Participant Items	Examples from Effective Interventions	Examples from Local Interventions (Write In)	Rating (Circle One)
1. The intervention meets specified priorities and needs defined by the community	Intervention sponsors social events for young men who have sex with men in communities that do not have places for them to congregate Intervention empowers peer volunteers to intervene in their own communities		High Medium Low
2. For the target population selected, the intervention is culturally competent	"Role model" stories used within the community are experiences of actual members of the community (with their names changed) English-Spanish video portrays real-life situations, decision-making processes, and condom negotiation strategies in appropriate Hispanic/Latino cultural context		High Medium Low
3. For the target population selected, the intervention is developmentally appropriate	The need for safer sex is introduced naturally into the casual conversations of mature adult men who have sex with men Runaway youth, ages 11 to 17, receive intervention messages in many entertaining ways and learn realistic expectations for skills development		High Medium Low
4. For the target population selected, the intervention is gender specific	An intervention targeting inner-city women is delivered by community women and focuses on women's health issues Young gay men receive an intervention through their social networks		High Medium Low
5. The intervention as implemented is acceptable to the participants	Participants continue to come, even without incentives Participants recommend the intervention to their friends		High Medium Low

Section 4
Appendices

Appendix A

HIV/AIDS Prevention Research Synthesis (PRS) Project Purpose and Selection Criteria

In 1996, CDC began the HIV/AIDS Prevention Research Synthesis (PRS) project to create a database of all HIV/AIDS behavioral, social, and policy studies to meet the needs of HIV prevention researchers, service providers and users, planners, policy makers, and others. The PRS project has several aims:

1) to conduct systematic reviews that address the population, intervention, study design, setting, and outcome factors associated with intervention effectiveness;

2) to identify methodologically rigorous studies that have statistically significant positive results; and

3) to identify gaps in the existing research and directions for future study.

The scope of the PRS project includes all studies with a focus on HIV prevention. Studies conducted in and outside the United States are included to enhance our understanding of risk reduction. Both published and unpublished reports of the studies are included to minimize the effect of "publication bias." Studies reported from 1988 onward are included in the database to coincide approximately with the start-up of HIV intervention research. A study typically was conducted two or three years earlier than the report date. The following types of studies are not considered part of our focus: biomedical-only, including vertical transmission; drug treatment only; occupational exposure; blood supply exposure; and referral-to-services-only.

Due to the time it takes to publish, index, and review studies, the PRS team, using the PRS database as of June 30, 1998, has reviewed about half of the studies reported or published between 1988-1996. The PRS team has not yet completed an extensive review of studies published or reported after 1996.

The PRS database and the Compendium will be updated periodically. At the time we completed the review for this Compendium, the PRS database contained approximately 4,000 citations on HIV prevention, which included 553 citations reporting on outcome evaluations of HIV risk reduction interventions. Among these, 276 studies were reviewed for PRS relevance and rigor criteria. Of the 276 intervention studies, 124 studies met all of the PRS criteria for relevance (measured at least one of the behavioral or biologic outcomes listed below) and methodologic rigor (used experimental or quasi-experimental designs with comparison groups). Of the remaining 152 intervention studies, 53 studies did not meet the PRS relevance criteria because they measured only psychosocial outcomes (Not Relevant) and 99 studies met the PRS relevance criteria but did not meet the criteria for methodologic rigor (Relevant Not Rigorous). The following describes in detail the PRS criteria for relevance and methodologic rigor, and Figure 1 illustrates the application of these criteria.

A. PRS Criteria

1. Criteria for Scope – These criteria are used to select studies that focus on HIV prevention interventions and that are not being studied extensively elsewhere. An in-scope study meets the following criteria:

(a) HIV prevention focus

(b) Reported from 1988 onward

(c) Published or unpublished

(d) Conducted inside or outside the U.S.

(e) Not drug treatment only

(f) Not biomedical only, (e.g., vaccine trials, AZT to prevent perinatal transmission)

(g) Not occupational exposure

(h) Not blood supply exposure

2. Criteria for Relevance – These criteria are used to select studies that aim to reduce sex- or drug-related risk behaviors or incidence rates of HIV or other STDs. The outcomes that PRS has determined to be relevant are those that directly impact the transmission of HIV or are indicators of HIV transmission. A relevant study must include one or more of the following outcomes:

Sex-related behaviors
- use of male condoms
- use of female condoms
- use of condom negotiation
- not having sex, if condom not used
- having unprotected sex
- number of sex partners
- mutually monogamous relationship
- partner selection
- return to abstinence
- initiation of first sexual intercourse
- exchanging sex for money/drugs

HIV testing behavior
- being tested
- learning test results
- repeat testing

Drug-related behaviors
- multi-person use of drug paraphernalia
- cleaning/bleaching drug paraphernalia
- use of new sterile needles/syringes
- injecting drugs
- initiation of drug injection
- non-injecting drug use
- sex with substance use
- return of used syringes

Health outcomes
- incidence rate of HIV, AIDS, STDs, HBV, or HCV
- prevalence rate of HIV, AIDS, STDs, HBV, or HCV

3. **Criteria for Methodologic Rigor** – All relevant studies are evaluated for methodologic rigor, regardless of the findings (i.e., studies with negative or null findings are included). These criteria are based on study design and vary by intervention category[1]. Behavioral and social intervention studies are classified as methodologically rigorous if they used random assignment to intervention and control groups (experimental designs) and reported at least post-intervention data. Behavioral and social studies are also considered rigorous if they used non-biased assignment (e.g., systematic assignment) to intervention and comparison groups (quasi-experimental designs) with equivalence of groups or used statistical adjustment for any nonequivalence, and reported pre- and post-intervention data. Policy interventions used these designs or less rigorous designs, such as designs with pre-post data but without a comparison group. These criteria are summarized below and in Figure 2.

(a) **For *behavioral and social* intervention studies:**

- Random assignment to intervention and comparison groups *WITH*
  - post-intervention data

- Non-random assignment to intervention and comparison groups using a non-biased method *WITH*
  - pre-post data *AND*
    - apparent equivalence of groups *OR*
    - adjustment for apparent non-equivalence of groups

(b) **For *policy* studies:**

- Random assignment to intervention and comparison groups *WITH*
  - post-intervention data

- Non-random assignment to intervention and comparison groups using a non-biased method, *WITH*
  - post-intervention data *AND*
    - apparent equivalence of groups *OR*
    - adjustment for apparent non-equivalence of groups

- Pre-post data with no comparison group

[1]There are three broad categories of interventions:

Behavioral interventions aim to change risk behaviors or decrease incidence rates of HIV or other sexually transmitted diseases (STDs). These tend to emphasize individual and small group approaches, e.g., counseling, small group discussion, skills demonstration.

Social interventions aim to change risk behaviors or decrease incidence rates of HIV or other STDs and also include explicit and direct attempts to change peer or community norms related to HIV risk. These interventions, while they may use individual or small group approaches, emphasize peer influence and community-level approaches, e.g., engaging key opinion leaders as educators and mobilizing the community to support HIV risk reduction behaviors. This category also includes any intervention aimed at changing environmental factors or structures related to HIV risk.

Policy studies aim to change risk behaviors or decrease incidence rates of HIV or STDs as a function of administrative or legal decisions, e.g., condom availability in public settings, HIV education in schools.

Figure A.1   PRS Review Process: Reviewed *OUTCOME STUDIES*, as of 6/30/98

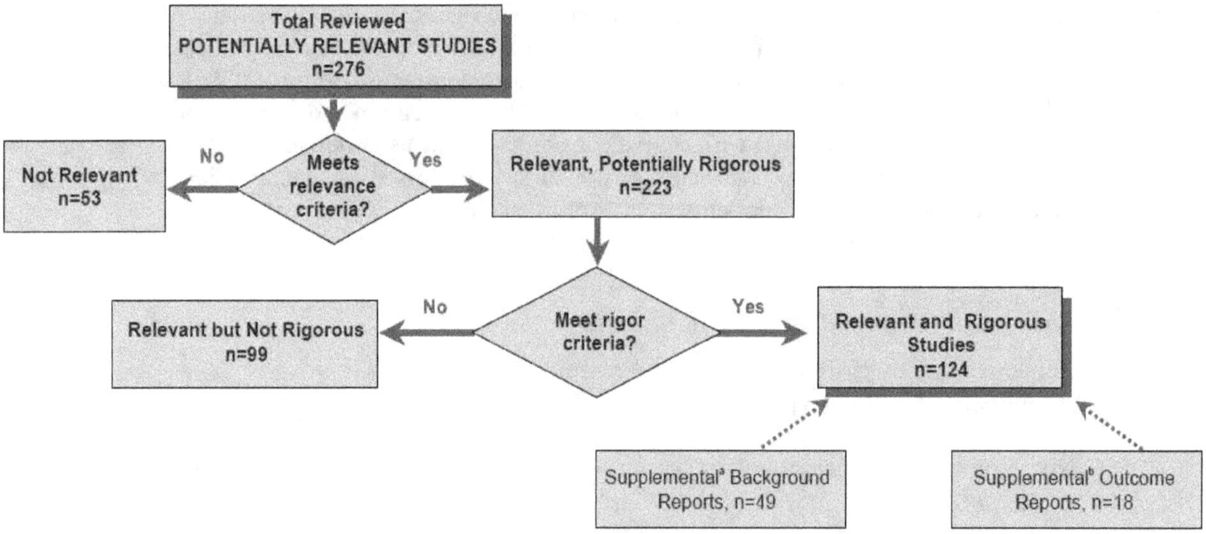

[a] Supplemental Background Reports provide information associated with primary studies, e.g. intervention description, methods baseline data
[b] Supplemental Outcome Reports provide evaluation data associated with primary studies, e.g. subsequent data waves, subsets of participants.

B. Compendium Criteria

To identify interventions for this *Compendium* we reviewed the *relevant and rigorous studies* using additional selection criteria:

1. **Studies conducted in the United States** – this Compendium is intended to meet the needs of prevention service providers, planners and others in the U.S., therefore, interventions conducted inside the U.S. were thought to be more applicable in context and content.

2. **Behavioral and social interventions, excluding policy studies** – Policy studies evaluate administrative or legislative decisions rather than an intervention per se. Most interventions that are the basis of a policy study have been evaluated elsewhere. For these reasons, only behavioral and social studies are included in this Compendium.

We then examined this subset, further selecting studies that met the following *effectiveness* criteria:

3. **Positive results on PRS relevant outcome(s)** – Outcomes that are relevant to PRS are those behaviors that would have a direct impact on HIV transmission and biological outcomes that are indicators of HIV transmission. Thus an important measure of a study's effectiveness is a positive result on at least one of these outcomes.

4. **Positive results that represent a statistically significant difference between the intervention and the control or comparison condition**

5. **No statistically significant negative findings on PRS relevant outcomes** – It would not be expedient to recommend an intervention that produced negative results for a behavior that directly impacts HIV transmission or for a biological indicator of HIV transmission, even though it may have produced a positive effect on another relevant behavior or indicator.

Figure A.2 illustrates the application of these criteria. Applying all five of these criteria resulted in the 24 interventions contained in this *Compendium*. Within the constraints indicated by the criteria listed above, these represent the best state-of-the-science interventions available as of June 30, 1998.

Consistent with these pre-established criteria, many studies were *not* selected for the *Compendium*. We did not select, for instance, studies where there was no control or comparison condition in the study design. Many of these studies with other designs provide valuable information but are out of the scope of this *Compendium*. Also, another CDC project, Characteristics of Reputationally Strong Programs (described elsewhere) examines such programs.

Figure A.2   Identify Effective Interventions

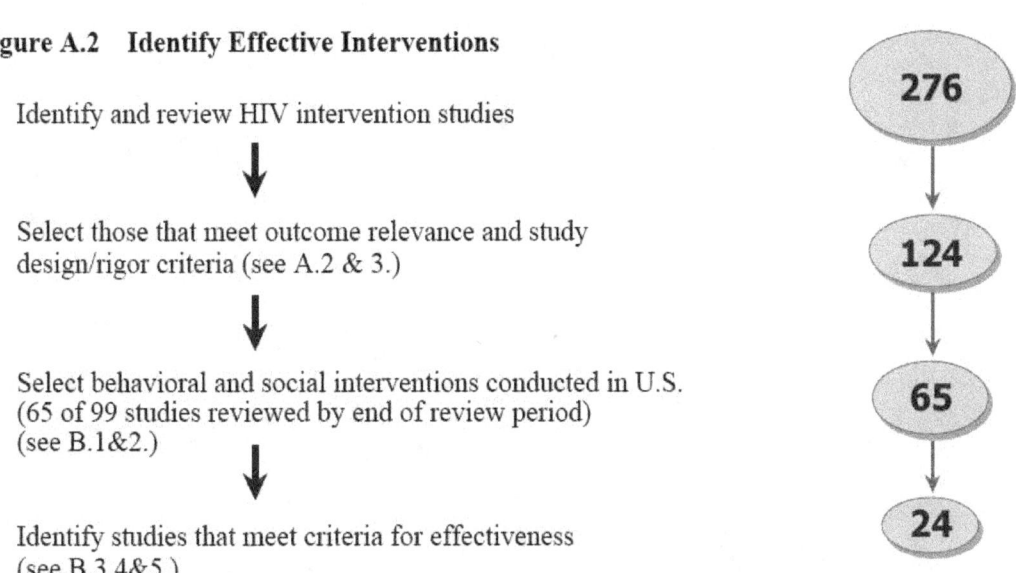

Identify and review HIV intervention studies

Select those that meet outcome relevance and study design/rigor criteria (see A.2 & 3.)

Select behavioral and social interventions conducted in U.S. (65 of 99 studies reviewed by end of review period) (see B.1&2.)

Identify studies that meet criteria for effectiveness (see B.3,4&5.)

276

124

65

24

---

[2] "Organizational Characteristics of Reputationally Strong Programs," Jane Mezoff, Brenda Seals, Ellen Sogolow, Bob Kohmescher, Gretchen Wooden, Larry Bye, Brian Tjugum, presented at the 12th World AIDS Conference, Geneva, June 28-July 3, 1998.

CDC's HIV/AIDS Prevention Research Synthesis Project, 404-639-1900, November 1999

Appendix B

Source Citations and Supplemental References

This appendix lists the source citations for the 24 intervention studies (★) described in this document. Additional or supplemental references are indented underneath the source citation for each intervention study. These additional references may be background citations (e.g., ones that contain descriptive information about the intervention) or outcome citations (e.g., ones that contain data from a subsequent follow-up assessment). These citations can help program planners obtain further information about the study design, methods, and other findings associated with the studies described in this document.

★CDC AIDS Community Demonstration Projects Research Group. (1999). Community-level HIV intervention in five cities: Final outcome data from the CDC AIDS Community Demonstration Projects. *American Journal of Public Health, 89* (3), 336-345.

Corby, N.H., & Wolitski, R.J., (Eds.). (1997). *Community HIV Prevention: The Long Beach AIDS Community Demonstration Project.* Long Beach, CA: The University Press, California State University, Long Beach.

Corby, N.H., Enguidandos, S.M., & Kay, L. (1996). Development and use of role-model stories in a community level HIV risk reduction intervention. *Public Health Reports, 111* (Supplement 1), 54-58.

Corby, N.H., & Wolitski, R. J. (1996). Condom use with main and other sex partners among high-risk women: Intervention outcomes and correlates of reduced risk. *Drugs and Society, 9* (1-2), 75-96.

Corby, N.H., Wolitski, R.J., Thorton-Johnson, S., & Tanner, W.M. (1991). AIDS knowledge, perception of risk, and behaviors among injection drug users. *AIDS Education and Prevention, 3* (4), 353-366.

Goldbaum, G., Perdue, T.R., & Higgins, D. (1996). Non-gay-identifying men who have sex with men: formative research results from Seattle, Washington. *Public Health Reports, 111* (Supplement 1), 36-40.

Goldbaum, G., Perdue, T., Wolitski, R., Rietmeijer, C., Hedrich, A., Wood, R., Fishbein, M., & the AIDS Community Demonstration Projects. (1998). Differences in risk behavior and sources of AIDS information among gay, bisexual, and straight-identified men who have sex with men. *AIDS and Behavior, 2* (1), 13-21.

Guenther-Grey, C.A., Tross, S., McAlister, A., Freeman, A., Cohn, D., Corby, N., Wood, R., & Fishbein, M. (1992). AIDS Community Demonstration Projects: Implementation of volunteer networks for HIV-prevention programs. *Morbidity and Mortality Weekly Report, 41*(46), 868-869, 875-876.

Higgins, D.L., O'Reilly, K., Tashima, N., Crain, C., Beeker, C., Goldbaum, G., Elifson, C.S., Galavotti, C., & Guenther-Gray, C. (1996). Using formative research to lay the foundation for community level HIV prevention efforts: An example from the AIDS Community Demonstration Projects. *Public Health Reports, 111* (Supplement 1), 28-35.

Krauss, B.J., Wolitski, R.J., Tross, S., Corby, N.H., & Fishbein, M. (Unpub.). *Getting the Message: HIV Information Sources of Women Who Have Sex With Injecting Drug Users: A Two-Site Study.* Atlanta, GA: Centers for Disease Control and Prevention.

Krepcho, M.A., Fernandez-Esquer, M.E., Freeman, A.C., Magee, E., & McAlister, A. (1993). Predictors of bleach use among current African-American injecting drug users: A community study. *Journal of Psychoactive Drugs, 25* (2), 135-141.

Krepcho, M.A., Smerick, M., Freeman, A., & Alfaro, A. (1993). Harnessing the energy of. the mass media: HIV awareness in Dallas. *American Journal of Public Health, 83*(2), 1-2.

O'Reilly, K.R., & Higgins, D. L. (1991). AIDS community demonstration projects for HIV, prevention among hard-to-reach groups. *Public Health Reports, 106* (6), 714-720.

Pulley, L., McAlister, A.L., Kay, L.S., & O'Reilly, K. (1996). Prevention campaigns for hard-to-reach populations at risk for HIV infection: Theory and implementation. *Health Education Quarterly, 23* (4), 488-496.

Rietmeijer, C. A., Kane, M. S., Simons, P. Z., Corby, N. H., Wolitski, R. J., Higgins, D. L., Judson, F. N., & Cohn, D. L. (1996). Increasing the use of bleach and condoms among injecting drug users in Denver: Outcomes of a targeted, community-level HIV prevention program. *AIDS, 10* (3), 291-298.

Schnell, D.J., Galavotti, C., & O'Reilly, K.R. (1993). An evaluation of sexual behaviour change using statistical and cognitive models. *Statistics in Medicine, 12*(3-4), 219-227.

Schnell, D.J., Magee, E., & Sheridan, J.R. (1995). A regression method for analysing ordinal data from intervention trials. *Statistics in Medicine, 14* (11), 1177-1189.

Simons, P.Z., Rietmeijer, C.A., Kane, M.S., Guenther-Grey, C., Higgins, D.L., & Cohn, D.L. (1996). Building a peer network for a community level HIV prevention program among injecting drug users in Denver. *Public Health Reports, 111* (Supplement 1), 50-53.

★Cohen, D., Dent, C., & MacKinnon, D. (1991). Condom skills education and sexually transmitted disease reinfection. *Journal of Sex Research, 28* (1), 139-144.

★Cohen, D.A., MacKinnon, D.P., Dent, C., Mason, H., & Sullivan, E. (1992). Group counseling at STD clinics to promote use of condoms. *Public Health Reports, 107* (6), 727-731.

★Des Jarlais, D.C., Casriel, C., Friedman, S.R., & Rosenblum, A. (1992). AIDS and the transition to illicit drug injection: Results of a randomized trial prevention program. *British Journal of Addiction, 87* (3), 493-498.

Casriel, C., Des Jarlais, D.C., Rodriguez, R., Friedman, S.R., Stepherson, B., & Khuri, E. (1990). Working with heroin sniffers: Clinical issues in preventing drug injection. *Journal of Substance Abuse Treatment, 7* (1), 1-10.

★DiClemente, R.J., & Wingood, G.M. (1995). A randomized controlled trial of an HIV sexual risk-reduction intervention for young African-American women. *Journal of the American Medical Association, 274* (16), 1271-1276.

★El-Bassel, N., & Schilling, R.F. (1992). 15-month follow-up of women methadone patients taught skills to reduce heterosexual HIV transmission. *Public Health Reports, 107* (5), 500-504.

Schilling, R.F., El-Bassel, N., Hadden, B., & Gilbert, L. (1995). Skills-training groups to reduce HIV transmission and drug use among methadone patients. *Social Work, 40* (1), 91-101.

★Hobfoll, S.E., Jackson, A.P., Lavin, J., Britton, P.J., & Shepherd, J.B. (1994). Reducing inner-city women's AIDS risk activities: A study of single, pregnant women. Health Psychology, *13* (5), 397-403.

★Jemmott, J.B., Jemmott, L.S., & Fong, G.T. (1992). Reductions in HIV risk-associated sexual behaviors among black male adolescents: Effects of an AIDS prevention intervention. *American Journal of Public Health, 82* (3), 372-377.

★Kamb, M.L., Fishbein, M., Douglas, J.M., Rhodes, F., Rogers, J., Bolan, G., Zenilman, J., Hoxworth, T., Malotte, C.K., Iatesta, M., Kent, C., Lentz, A., Graziano, S., Byers, R.H., & Peterman, T.A., for the Project RESPECT Study Group. (1998). Efficacy of risk-reduction counseling to prevent Human Immunodeficiency Virus and sexually transmitted diseases: A randomized controlled trial. *Journal of the American Medical Association, 280* (13), 1161-1167.

★Kegeles, S.M., Hays, R.B., & Coates, T.J. (1996). The Mpowerment Project: A community-level HIV prevention intervention for young gay men. *American Journal of Public Health, 86* (8), 1129-1136.

★Kelly, J.A., Murphy, D.A., Washington, C.D., Wilson, T.S., Koob, J.J., Davis, D.R., Ledezma, G., & Davantes, B. (1994). The effects of HIV/AIDS intervention groups for high-risk women in urban clinics. *American Journal of Public Health, 84* (12), 1918-1922.

Holtgrave, D.F., & Kelly, J.A. (1996). Preventing HIV/AIDS among high-risk urban women: The cost-effectiveness of a behavioral group intervention. *American Journal of Public Health, 86* (10), 1442-1445.

Vander Linden, C. (1993). NIMH prevention research helps women change AIDS risk behavior. *Public Health Reports, 108* (3), 413.

★Kelly, J.A., St. Lawrence, J.S., Diaz, Y.E., Stevenson, L.Y., Hauth, A.C., Brasfield, T.L., Kalichman, S.C., Smith, J.E., & Andrew, M.E. (1991). HIV risk behavior reduction following intervention with key opinion leaders of population: An experimental analysis. *American Journal of Public Health, 81* (2), 168-171.

Kelly, J.A. (1994). Sexually transmitted disease prevention approaches that work: Interventions to reduce risk behavior among individuals, groups, and communities. *Sexually Transmitted Diseases, 21* (2, Suppl.), S73-S75.

Kelly, J.A., St. Lawrence, J.S., Stevenson, Y., Hauth, A.C., Kalichman, S.C., Diaz, Y.E., Brasfield, T.L., Koob, J.J., & Morgan, M.G. (1992). Community AIDS/HIV risk reduction: The effects of endorsements by popular people in three cities. *American Journal of Public Health, 82* (11), 1483-1489.

Pinkerton, S.D., Holtgrave, D.R., DiFranceisco, W.J., Stevenson, L.Y., & Kelly, J.A. (1998). Cost-effectiveness of a community-level HIV risk reduction intervention. *American Journal of Public Health, 88* (8), 1239-1242.

★Kelly, J.A., St. Lawrence, J.S., Hood, H.V., & Brasfield, T.L. (1989). Behavioral intervention to reduce AIDS risk activities. *Journal of Consulting and Clinical Psychology, 57* (1), 60-67.

★Kirby, D., Barth, R.P., Leland, N., & Fetro, J.V. (1991). Reducing the risk: Impact of a new curriculum on sexual risk-taking. *Family Planning Perspectives, 23* (6), 253-263.

★Lauby, J., Smith, P.J.,Stark, M., Person, B., & Adams, J. (2000). A community-level HIV prevention intervention for inner city women: Results of the Women and Infants Demonstration Projects. *American Journal of Public Health, 90* (2), 216-222.

    Bond, L., Bowden-Proctor, J., Lauby, J., Walls, C. & Woll, M. (1997). Developing non-traditional print media for HIV prevention: Role model stories for young urban women. *American Journal of Public Health, 87* (2), 289-290.

    Lauby, J.L., Semaan, S., Cohen, A., Leviton, L., Gielen, A., Pulley, L., Walls, C., & O'Campo, P. (1998). Self-efficacy, decisional balance and stages of change for condom use among women at risk for HIV infection. *Health Education Research, 13* (3), 343-356.

    Person, B., Cotton, D., & Prevention of HIV in Women and Infants Demonstration Projects. (1996). Model of community mobilization for the prevention of HIV in women and infants. *Public Health Reports, 111*(Supplement 1), 89-98.

    Terry, M.A., Liebman, J., Person, B., Bond, L., Dillard-Smith, C., & Tunstall, C. (1999). Women and Infants Demonstration Project: An integrated approach to AIDS prevention and research. *AIDS Education and Prevention, 11* (2), 107-121.

★Magura, S., Kang, S., & Shapiro, J.L. (1994). Outcomes of intensive AIDS education for male adolescent drug users in jail. *Journal of Adolescent Health, 15* (6), 457-463.

★Main, D.S., Iverson, D.C., McGloin, J., Banspach, S.W., Collins, J.L., Rugg, D.L., & Kolbe, L.J. (1994). Preventing HIV infection among adolescents: Evaluation of a school-based education program. *Preventive Medicine, 23* (4), 409-417.

★McCusker, J., Stoddard, A.M., Zapka, J.G., Morrison, C.S., Zorn, M., & Lewis, B.F. (1992). AIDS education for drug abusers: Evaluation of short-term effectiveness. *American Journal of Public Health, 82* (4), 533-540.

★O'Donnell, C.R., O'Donnell, L., San Doval, A., Duran, R., & Labes, K. (1998). Reductions in STD infections subsequent to an STD clinic visit: Using video-based patient education to supplement provider interactions. *Sexually Transmitted Diseases, 25* (3), 161-168.

O'Donnell, C.R., O'Donnell, L., San Doval, A., Duran, R., & Labes, K. (1994). *Clinic -based research and demonstration project to prevent sexually transmitted disease among high risk blacks and Latinos: The efficacy of video-based education in reducing STD infections subsequent to an STD clinic visit.* (Final Report). Newton, MA: Education Development Center, Inc.

O'Donnell, L.N., San Doval, A., Duran, R., & O'Donnell, C.R. (1995). The effectiveness of video-based interventions in promoting condom acquisition among STD clinic patients. *Sexually Transmitted Diseases* 22 (2), 97-103.

★Rotheram-Borus, M.J., Van Rossem, R., Gwadz, M., Koopman, C., & Lee, M. (1997). *Reductions in HIV risk among runaway youths.* Los Angeles, CA: University of California, Department of Psychiatry, Division of Social and Community Psychiatry.

Rotheram-Borus, M.J., Koopman, C., Haignere, C., & Davies, M. (1991). Reducing HIV sexual risk behaviors among runaway adolescents. *Journal of the American Medical Association, 266* (9), 1237-1241.

★St. Lawrence, J.S., Brasfield, T.L., Jefferson, K.W., Alleyne, E., O'Bannon, R.E., & Shirley, A. (1995). Cognitive-behavioral intervention to reduce African American adolescents' risk for HIV infection. *Journal of Consulting and Clinical Psychology, 63* (2), 221-237.

★Stanton, B.F., Li, X., Ricardo, I., Galbraith, J., Feigelman, S., & Kaljee, L. (1996). A randomized, controlled effectiveness trial of an AIDS prevention program for low-income African-American youths. *Archives of Pediatrics and Adolescent Medicine, 150* (4), 363-372.

Stanton, B., Fang, X., Li, X., Feigelman, S., Galbraith, J., & Ricardo, I. (1997). Evolution of risk behaviors over 2 years among a cohort of urban African American adolescents. *Archives of Pediatrics and Adolescent Medicine, 151* (4), 398-406.

★Valdiserri, R.O., Lyter, D.W., Leviton, L.C., Callahan, C.M., Kingsley, L.A., & Rinaldo, C.R. (1989). AIDS prevention in homosexual and bisexual men: Results of a randomized trial evaluating two risk reduction interventions. *AIDS, 3* (1), 21-26.

★Wenger, N.S., Linn, L.S., Epstein, M., & Shapiro, M.F. (1991). Reduction of high-risk sexual behavior among heterosexuals undergoing HIV antibody testing: A randomized control trial. *American Journal of Public Health, 81* (12), 1580-1585.